SCOLIOSIS
ASCENDING THE CURVE

SCOLIOSIS
ASCENDING
THE CURVE

BROOKE LYONS with

OHENEBA BOACHIE-ADJEI, M.D.,

JOHN PODZIUS, PH.D.,

and CARLA PODZIUS, CSW

M. Evans and Company, Inc.
New York

M. Evans and Company, Inc.
216 East 49th Street
New York, New York 10017

Library of Congress Cataloging-in-Publication Data

Lyons, Brooke.
    Scoliosis : ascending the curve / by Brooke Lyons with Oheneba Boachie-Adjei, John Podzius, and Carla Podzius.
        p.   cm.
    ISBN 0-87131-883-0
    1. Scoliosis Popular works. 2. Spine—Abnormalities. 3. Scoliosis—Psychological aspects. I. Boachie-Adjei, Oheneba, 1950–   II. Podzius, John. III. Podzius, Carla. IV. Title.
RD771.S3L98   1999
616.7'3—dc21   99-28380

Book design and typesetting by Rik Lain Schell

Printed in the United States of America

9 8 7 6 5 4 3 2 1

ASK YOUR DOCTOR

This book does not substitute for the medical advice and supervision of your personal physician. While the advice in this book comes from the experience of a scoliosis patient, a scoliosis surgeon, and a psychologist, no book can substitute for the relationship between patient and doctor. Scoliosis should always be treated by trained medical personnel who are aware of the most current developments in this changing field.

Contents

To Janice Sacks, who, instead of allowing her lifelong bout with scoliosis to hinder her, allowed it only to impel her toward triumph and happiness. We can relate to Janice's story, we can learn from her experience, and we can benefit from her energy, her generosity, and her strength. Janice's devotion to bolstering scoliosis awareness is outshined only by her infectious determination and her tireless concern for others. To convey all that Janice Sacks embodies is the goal, ambitious though it may be, of this book.

Acknowledgments

First and foremost, I would like to thank the people whom I interviewed for this book. I am sure you will find their stories and their words of wisdom intriguing and inspiring, just as I did. In particular, I thank Sherry, Sylvia, James Blake, Pat, Sabina, Denise, Linda, Jeanette Lee, Sondra, Anthony, Michelle Mauney, Erika, Kelly Patten, Eric, Marianne, Jennifer, Alison, Charlie, David, Wendy Whelan, and Zoe, whose provoking stories constitue the fabric of this book.

Many, many thanks to my editor, Nancy Hancock, without whom my vision of a scoliosis book would never have come to fruition. Nancy, you believed in me, you taught me the ways of the literary world, you collaborated with me, and you spent hundreds of hours fine-tuning my book; I am forever grateful to you.

I would also like to thank Dr. Oheneba Boachie-Adjei, Dr. John Podzius, and Carla Podzius for their insightful contributions to this project. Dr. Boachie, John, and Carla, I am indebted to you, and I thank you for your vast knowledge, your generous assistance, and your hard work.

Thank you to Kenneth Hopkins, who traveled with me to a number of locations and managed to shoot beautiful photographs in settings ranging from a penthouse to a horse farm. Ken, thank you for your creativity, your many talents, your loyalty, and your friendship.

Many thanks to Janice and Stanley Sacks, who trusted me, when I was fourteen years old, to establish a local chapter of the national scoliosis support group they run. They opened my eyes to a world of knowledge and compassion; they taught me virtually everything I know about scoliosis; and they altered the path of my life.

I must thank Diana Zitnay and Jennifer Bloomgarden for repeatedly rescuing me from my computer woes; Dr. Tushar Ch. Patel for providing me with a firsthand look at scoliosis surgery; Victor Trevino for putting me in touch with Ms. Whelan; Ann Wallin for constantly giving me words of advice and encouragement; and Mary Bennett and Carolyn Spann-Vega for being some of the most helpful resources in Dr. Boachie's office.

Finally, I thank my parents, Penny and Jim Lyons, for their tremendous support of all my endeavors, and my siblings, Blake and Chloe, for putting up with me during the various stages of this book's production. Thank you to all of my friends from Hopkins, particularly Zoë Klugman, who understood my being "busy with the book" for two years and who remained patient and supportive. And thank you to everyone at the New England Ballet for their interest in scoliosis and their enthusiasm for raising scoliosis awareness.

Foreword

Scoliosis is a multifaceted problem, but is often written about as only an explanation of the spinal deformity and resulting treatment. However, the full scope of physical, psychological, and social issues must be recognized by the patient, physician, and family if an effective integration of treatment and lifestyle is to be achieved. This book provides information and inspiration to help scoliosis patients and their families rise above the complexities of scoliosis.

It is obvious that scoliosis is first and foremost a physical spinal deformity. The physical aspects of scoliosis can be alarming to a newly diagnosed patient. The physical problems and limitations of a scoliotic deformity can be overwhelming.

The psychological impact of scoliosis, often unrecognized, can bring negative self-esteem, intense feelings of rejection, and isolation from family and friends. Many times the diagnosis of scoliosis in an adolescent, compounded by the need for wearing a brace and special clothing to cover it, and peer group pressure, can be traumatic. There is an intense preoccupation with body image. Parents and families can be an infinite source of support and positive reinforcement, but many feel unsure of the best approach. Other psychological aspects come into play as the recommendation of surgery becomes a reality. Children and adolescents often take their cues in coping from observing the parent's reaction. Fear and anxiety related to the procedure, the outcome, and the resulting scar can easily be projected from parent to child.

Adult scoliosis patients find that chronic pain compounded by disc degeneration, sciatica, spinal stenosis, and arthritic changes in the joints and vertebrae can torment a life. The debilitating effects of scoliosis bring new challenges and require appropriate evaluation and clearminded decision making. Often, adults with scoliosis have more medical problems than teenagers. Additionally, they may feel isolated in coping and decision making, often lacking the understanding of family and friends.

This book addresses all aspects of living with scoliosis. Whether you are the patient or a family member, you will find helpful advice, useful information, and positive direction. Throughout the book you will find inspiring, informative stories from individuals and families touched by scoliosis.

Brooke Lyons, president of the Scoliosis Association of Connecticut and the national teen spokesperson for the Scoliosis Association, Inc., realized the need for this informative and enlightening book for the scoliosis patient, general public, and health professional. Oheneba Boachie-Adjei, M.D., chief of scoliosis surgery at the Hospital for Special Surgery in New York City, has provided the medical expertise for this encompassing book. John Podzius, Ph.D., clinical psychologist, and Carla Podzius, M.S.W., have contributed their experience and knowledge concerning the emotional and social stresses of scoliosis.

When Brooke first contacted our national organization at the age of fourteen, she sought support and information about her own scoliosis and was dismayed that there was no chapter in her area. She proceeded to found the Connecticut chapter, reaching outward to others by establishing a toll-free hotline. Brooke spent many hours listening to and counseling other teens and parents on compliance in bracewear and other concerns. She organized and conducted meetings, publicized her chapter in the media, and arranged for noted professionals to speak at chapter meetings. Brooke was committed to providing increased public awareness of scoliosis. She educated herself by reading everything available on the subject and spoke to nurses involved with school screening programs. Brooke also conducted events to raise over $15,000 for scoliosis research, again raising public awareness. She has received national honors for her dedication and volunteerism in the community, and for furthering greater public awareness of scoliosis. She is a dynamic young woman who provides a powerful influence for other teenagers. Her commitment, perseverance, and dedication to finding the cause of scoliosis and helping others cope with its challenges should be a paradigm for other patients and families. She has accomplished so much at such a young age. We are proud to acknowledge the gargantuan achievement of writing this educational, informative, and inspirational book.

Stanley E. Sacks, President
Janice T. Sacks, Executive Vice President
The Scoliosis Association, Inc.

An Unexpected Curve in Fate's Path

Some people believe that all beings are endowed, at birth, with particular and immutable fates. Other people claim that all beings have the inherent power to determine their fates. The debate over predestination has, for centuries, permeated life, literature, and culture. I am one of the many people who relish exploring the vast realms of such questions. Ever since I have been old enough to understand the meaning of fate, I have been fascinated by its debatable existence and its indeterminate power. I have found the concept of fate to be frightening yet comforting, perplexing yet intriguing, and disappointing yet promising.

I used to think that I could rule my own fate. Far from being idealistic, this belief was appropriate, for every aspect of my life, at that point, had been planned, expected, and welcomed. My life resembled a straight path which, when I peered down it, continued infinitely in the same direction.

I am now able to see how inane my perception of life used to be. This realization fell upon me when, during the summer before my freshman year in high school, I was jolted by a sudden curve in my life's otherwise straight path. That summer I attended the Boston Ballet Summer Dance Program, one of the finest programs in the country. Feeling privileged to be one of two hundred students chosen from sixteen hundred who auditioned, I worked very hard at perfecting my ballet skills, often dancing up to five hours per day. On weekends, my parents traveled to Boston to visit. Seeing and hearing about how fatigued my body was from all the dancing, they treated me to a massage. As I eagerly entered the massage room I expected to meet a masseuse, but the woman I met was, instead, a physiotherapist. Her credentials enabled her to explain details about muscles, bones, tendons, and body alignment as she performed the massage.

Her expert hands seemed magical in their ability to relax my muscles and mitigate my aching, and her abundant yet soft-spoken words were greatly informative. When her hands reached my back, she suddenly exclaimed, "Wow!"

"What?" I asked.

"You have bad scoliosis, don't you?" she asked back.

"What?" I asked again.

"You know," she answered, "scoliosis." But I didn't know.

"Your spine is curved," she explained.

"Really? That's strange," I replied, laughing nervously. At that point, I had no idea what the implications of the woman's discovery would be.

Following the massage the physiotherapist—who, knowing more about my situation that I knew, was more concerned than I was—explained her findings to my parents. Calmly, they said they would make an appointment for me to see an orthopedic surgeon when I returned from Boston.

Within the next month, I had seen three specialists in scoliosis. My mind turned into a kaleidoscope of hospital and doctor names, complex medical jargon, and various diagnoses. In the midst of the confusion, I desperately wondered what was happening to me. Why, I wondered, had this aberration come to afflict not only my spine, but my life as well?

My first visit was to a scoliosis surgeon who quite bluntly said, "You have moderately severe scoliosis. I can't believe that it has remained unnoticed for so long." My mother and I gazed at the full length X ray of my body, which brightly illuminated a spine in the shape of a backward letter "S." Surely, I thought, that can't be my spine. There must be some mistake. How could I possibly walk, much less dance? The surgeon continued talking in a very robotic manner. "You have a double major curve measuring thirty degrees and thirty-six degrees. You are too old to brace since you are probably finished growing. I recommend that you have surgery. Surgery will consist of a spinal fusion, with two steel rods inserted into the spine. You probably won't be able to continue with your dancing after that. But don't worry. After a year of healing, you'll be able to function just as any *normal* person would. You will be able to do activities like swimming, soccer, softball, tennis, running. Do you have any questions?"

Well, yes, I did have questions, but all I could do was sit there silently. My mind was too numb to produce words for me to speak. It would be two more weeks until my next appointment with another scoliosis specialist. My world took on a grim character as the winds of fate forced me around the sharp curves of the new dark and torturous path. My newfound scoliosis and its implications swiftly buried the ballet slippers, flowers, and days of perfect health that had previously paved my way. I soon became painfully aware of man's pathetic ineptitude to control fate and of fate's formidable ability to control man.

While the definitive diagnosis shocked and upset me, it also made me think about the past and the tremendous role ballet had played in my life. At the age of fourteen I had been dancing for about eleven years. When I was thirteen years old and in the seventh grade, my ballet teacher at a local school in Connecticut told my mother it was time to take me to New York.

"She has the potential to make it as a dancer," he said. The following year, I traveled an hour and a half to New York City four nights each week and attended ballet classes at the Joffrey Ballet School.

After dancing almost every evening at a famous ballet school in New York, participating in various ballet performances throughout the year, and maintaining straight A's in school, I boldly decided that I would, after high school, attend a competitive university and dance in a nearby professional dance company. I saw myself steering a boat in the ocean of fate toward a definite, promising future. Yet that next summer not only was I removed from the steering position, but I was thrown from the ship. Now helpless against fate's current, I floated unwillingly toward some unknown destiny.

I suddenly found myself back in Boston—only this time, on the other side of the city at the Boston Children's Hospital. The juxtaposition of the ballet metropolis, with girls and boys hustling to class and exercising and stretching in the hallways, to children in wheelchairs surrounded by sad parents, most with a look of desperation or resignation, was jolting. This orthopedic surgeon was much more thorough in his approach. He suggested an X ray of my hand to determine my exact bone age and bending X rays to see how much flexibility I had in my spine. "If you are not fully grown, I would recommend bracing at this point to give yourself every opportunity to avoid surgery," he said. "If the X rays show that you are fully grown, I would recommend not bracing and waiting an additional six months to see if there is a progression of your curves. If you progress after you are fully grown, you will most likely become a candidate for a spinal fusion to halt the progression." And then, he addressed the single most important point without provocation. "About your ballet. . . ," he began. He told me that while I would be able to dance *recreationally,* my dreams of dancing professionally were no longer realistic and I would no longer be able to perform due to the loss of flexibility. Diminished flexibility means diminished ability. I couldn't hold back the tears that ran down my face as the doctor asked, "Do you have any questions?" Finally, I found my voice.

"Wait a minute," I said. "I *can't* have a spinal fusion and lose the flexibility in my back. Ballet is one of the most important aspects of my life, and I will never give it up. What will happen if I opt never to have surgery?"

Slowly the doctor replied, "The curves can progress one to two degrees per year, which is the generally accepted rate of progression. The spine will continue to curve and rotate. As the spine twists, the ribs will twist causing, in the more advanced cases, compression of the organs, possibly leading to heart problems and diminished lung capacity. Aesthetically, if left untreated, a progressive scoliosis could give one a hunchback-like appearance. Scoliosis takes time to progress. It could be several years before you need surgery, and you might not have any major physical problems at all."

I knew, at that point, that surgery was inevitable; I drifted defenselessly along with fate's current.

In the waiting room of the X-ray department, I found myself surrounded by burned children with terribly contracted scars and children with missing limbs and prostheses. I was startled when the X-ray technician called my name. As I walked into the X-ray room, I realized that during that brief waiting period I was completely immersed in the conditions of those around me, fascinated by their ability to smile, to converse with their parents and with each other. Suddenly, my condition paled by comparison.

We returned to the scoliosis clinic nervously awaiting the results of my X rays. My empty gaze wandered to a bulletin board filled with letters from kids who had had scoliosis surgery. Some talked of their ninety-five-degree curves and how happy they were with their corrections. Many offered their names and addresses to answer questions. The letters were warmly written and filled with sincere gratitude, hope, and appreciation for their straighter spines. I was awestruck. As the hours of this day went by, I began to feel slightly less heavyhearted.

Summoned back into the examining room, I met with the news that I still had fifteen months of growth left and that I *was* braceable. I was so happy to hear that! Even better was the news that if surgery was necessary in the future, it would probably only be in the thoracic area (located within or involving the thorax), thus allowing me to maintain most of my flexibility. Performing, however, would still not be a possibility.

It was recommended that we seek treatment closer to home for convenience. My third opinion was from an orthopedic surgeon from Columbia Presbyterian in New York City who completely concurred with the orthopedic surgeon from Boston Children's Hospital. The next weeks were filled with visiting the orthotist for brace consultation and fitting.

The murky waters began to clear up. I asked questions and talked to anyone who looked like a possible resource. The more I educated myself, the more control I felt over my destiny. I would happily wear my brace and hope that it would halt the progression of my curves.

The brace fitting was filled with laughter, awkwardness, and terror! A stockingette was placed over my body like a tight sheath dress. They wrapped me with four-inch gauze in mummy-like fashion and wet down my entire body. I felt so silly and uncomfortable! My mom and I were laughing uncontrollably after the orthotist left the room while "I dried." When it had completely hardened, he returned to cut it off with a saw—a terrifying experience. The saw never came close to my body, however. Two weeks later, we returned to receive this work of art. I sported a cotton t-shirt (my undergarment for the next year) and tried on my new fashion statement. Adjustments were made to this custom-molded, low-profile brace to ensure maximum comfort and, of course, maximum compliance. I would return every month thereafter for an adjustment of the pads inside that would provide just the right amount of pressure to keep my spine from curving more.

My brace was to become my new best friend. Although it was very hot, tight, and uncomfortable and caused me some sleepless nights, I was religious about wearing it the prescribed eighteen hours per day, taking it off only for showers and my daily dance classes. It eventually became like just another part of my body. After a few months, I didn't even know I had it on.

As I turned fifteen, I got a new wardrobe of oversized clothes and off I went to begin high school with braces on my teeth and a brace on my body! There was only one way to deal with it, and that was to be very open and explain to everyone why I looked a little strange. The kids were wonderfully accepting of it, oftentimes jokingly punching "my abs of steel (or plastic)!"

By being very open about having scoliosis and not ashamed to wear or talk about my brace, I eliminated the possibility of having people talk about it behind my back. I made people comfortable talking about it right in front of me, and this acceptance of my brace I found very pleasing. I think that if you accept your scoliosis for what it is, and maintain and exude a confident attitude, there is nothing to be afraid of.

Though I quickly became more comfortable with my situation, I still had many unanswered questions. With limited local resources, I sought the support of the Scoliosis Association, Inc., a national support and information organization. The nearest chapter was an hour and a half away in Long Island. My parents and I traveled to attend a meeting and found it helpful to meet people with whom there was a common bond. My attitude toward fate and toward scoliosis underwent a major transformation. I vividly remembered how isolated, sad, and helpless I had felt upon discovering my scoliosis, and I also vividly remembered the letters on the bulletin board. In hopes of preventing others from having to go through the same painful mental process that I went through, I established the first Connecticut Chapter of the Scoliosis Association, Inc. With the support of Janice and Stanley Sacks, president and vice-president of the national organization, and of my family, my chapter became a positive force in my life and the lives of others.

A year later, my curves had basically held, only progressing to thirty-six degrees and thirty-nine degrees. The doctor told me I was "almost" finished growing and that I didn't need to bring the brace to France with me that summer, where I would study ballet at Le Centre de Danse International in Cannes. Again, we would wait and see. Six months later my X rays revealed a progression of my curves to forty degrees and forty-two degrees. I was told to return in one year. At this point, two years had passed from the time of diagnosis. During the summer before my junior year in high school, X rays revealed a progression to forty-nine degrees and fifty-one degrees, necessitating surgery "within the next year." Again, I sought three opinions, only this time to determine the surgical approach. All three opinions differed. How does one make a choice? My choice was made based on education about and involvement with scoliosis, my lifestyle, and, most importantly, my gut reaction to the person I would come to call my surgeon.

As the time for my surgery draws nearer, I'm neither nervous nor sad. At this point, I've had plenty of time to sort out the hand that fate dealt me. Even with my calm, accepting attitude toward my scoliosis surgery, however, as the days pass I feel the final vestiges of my dancing dreams being torn from my soul. For the past few years, living and dancing with scoliosis has been a fact of my life. After the surgery, however, living and, perhaps, attempting to dance with metal hooks and rods lodged in my spine will undoubtedly be an even harsher reality to face.

Now, a senior in high school, I am embracing my last dance performances as I busy myself preparing for college and looking to a new future. Myriad experiences over the past three years as president and founder of the Scoliosis Association of Connecticut and as the National Teen Spokesperson for the Scoliosis Association, Inc., have taught me that my path in life is not, in fact, as doomed as it seemed to be on the day of my diagnosis. I now realize that, while scoliosis is a debilitating condition, it is treatable; and that, while scoliosis has caused a complete upheaval in my life, it has reciprocated by teaching me valuable lessons. Through many blessings, I have been fortunate to turn the negative impact of having scoliosis into a positive—though bittersweet—opportunity. I have gained invaluable amounts of strength, optimism, perspective, and life experience.

I once thought that I could control fate. Then I was convinced that fate controlled me. I now believe that fate and man are equally responsible for determining the path of a life. The story of one's life is neither a blank piece of paper nor a finished work of literature; it is, rather, a rough draft. To write the rough draft is fate's duty; to augment and edit fate's draft is the duty of the individual living the story.

Having been assigned the wonderous task of editing my own particular rough draft, I have decided to put all of my effort into making it a masterpiece. Why be miserable when you can be happy? Life is never perfect; unfortunate circumstances inevitably arise. Only by working patiently, constructively, and creatively with whatever rough draft fate puts forth can the entitled produce the exceptional work of literature, what all individuals worldwide strive for—a fulfilling life.

CHAPTER 1

WHAT IS SCOLIOSIS?

So! What is scoliosis? Is it a disease? No. Is it a disorder? Yes. A deformity? Yes. A growth deviation? Yes. Why do we have it? Possibly genetics; research seems to be pointing in that direction. Scoliosis was, until recently, defined as a lateral curvature of the spine. Today, scoliosis is more accurately defined as a three-dimensional curvature of the spine. While the lateral curvature of patients' spines continues to remain important, the rotation of patients' spines has become a more crucial and widely recognized issue than it previously was. A great amount of lateral curvature in the spine causes some physical deformity (*i.e.,* an inclination to bend or slouch to one side or a noticeable crease in the waist) and tends to make X rays look more dramatic. A great amount of rotation, on the other hand, can affect patients in both appearance and health. Since the spine is connected to the rib cage, rotation of the spine causes a corresponding rotation of the rib cage; this rotation can be seen in the rib humps that develop in most scoliosis patients. The more the rib cage is rotated, the more it compresses the organs within its realms. As a result of severe rotation of the spine, therefore, some patients develop heart problems or experience decreases in their lung capacities. Nevertheless, these implications of rotation apply only to those patients whose thoracic curves have progressed to measurements of about sixty-five or more degrees and vary according to each individual patient's health.

Scoliosis is more prevalent in our society than most people imagine. But many people with scoliosis have such a minimal degree of curvature that its presence can go unnoticed. People with scoliosis requiring treatment can feel as though they are alone in having the disorder. Statistics supporting the actual prevalence of scoliosis in today's society should convince every scoliosis patient that they are in no way alone. There are twenty-five scoliosis cases per one thousand people (1/40th of the population) for curves of at least ten degrees; for scoliosis curves greater than twenty degrees, the prevalence drops to three to five cases per one thousand people (at most, 1/200th of the population); and for curves greater than thirty degrees, the prevalence is only one to three cases per one thousand people (at most, 1/333rd of the population). Unfortunately for females, the female-to-male ratio for curves greater than ten degrees is two to one; for curves greater than twenty degrees, the ratio increases to five to one; and for curves greater than thirty degrees, the ratio is a whopping ten to one. For some unknown reason, females are much more likely to develop scoliosis than males. Many females find this news to be both upsetting and unfair, yet it is irrefutable. I strongly suggest that anyone who has scoliosis promptly recognize the challenge and make choices that will bring about long-term health and well-being. In order to gain the confidence necessary to face scoliosis, I encourage an approach that combines optimism, honesty, and bravery. Try to gain solace from knowing that others are facing the same daily challenges and finding positive ways to cope with and overcome physical limitations.

No single description of scoliosis can encompass the wide range of scoliosis curves that exist. Variables such as the origin of scoliosis, the time of the onset of scoliosis, the location of the curve, the degree of curvature, and the behavior of the curve provide a foundation for any number of scoliosis cases. Because scoliosis can manifest itself in many different ways, doctors must classify scoliosis cases before they can assess and recommend a treatment for a particular case. The categorization of scoliosis is usually decided according to the curve's shape, cause, location, and severity.

The shape of a curve is determined by its unique combination of lateral curvature and rotation. Some curves present considerable lateral curvature and an insignificant amount of rotation; some, on the other hand, exhibit much rotation and little lateral curvature. Still others are characterized by severe lateral curvature and severe rotation. Physical symptoms of scoliosis and suggested scoliosis treatments are dependent upon the combination of lateral curvature and rotation that a particular curve displays.

In terms of causes of scoliosis, an important distinction lies between structural scoliosis and functional, or nonstructural, scoliosis. Structural scoliosis is caused by the natural progression of one's spine into a curved position. It cannot be fixed by merely sitting and standing up straight; it is a natural and often irrevocable force that requires proactive treatment. Comparatively, functional scoliosis is the result of muscular or gravitational pull on the spine and is often caused by activities such as chronic slouching, resting a baby on the same hip each time you hold him or her, or carrying a bag or backpack on one shoulder all the time. It may take years for functional scoliosis to develop; once it has developed, it can be corrected by stretching and toning one's back, making a conscientious effort to sit and stand up straight, or wearing an informal sort of back brace (not necessarily one designed particularly for scoliosis patients). Irritative lesions such as disc herniation or tumor of the spine can cause structural scoliosis, which can spontaneously correct after the irritative lesion is removed.

All structural scoliosis cases can be placed in either one of two categories: the idiopathic cases, and the cases that are related to an identifiable reason or condition. *Idiopathic* means that there is no known cause of the scoliosis; it simply appears in the patient's spine and is unrelated to anything else. Eighty-five percent of all people with scoliosis have the idiopathic type, and, despite extensive research, the actual cause of idiopathic scoliosis remains unknown.[1] Of the eighty-five percent of scoliosis cases that are idiopathic, the female-to-male ratio of incidence is seven to one (for reasons presently unknown to researchers, doctors, and patients). Scoliosis of a known origin is usually the result of a neuromuscular disease or a congenital abnormality.

Not only can scoliosis be divided into categories according to origin, but it can be categorized by the time (in a patient's life) at which it appears. Congenital scoliosis normally originates when there is an abnormal formation of the spine or spinal cord while the child is just an embryo. It may be present at birth or develop shortly after. Congenital scoliosis tends to affect equal numbers of males and females and to pose a twenty to thirty percent higher risk for spinal cord abnormalities than idiopathic scoliosis does. The two main reasons for

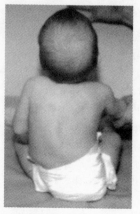 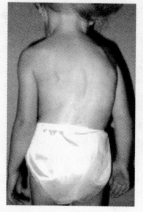 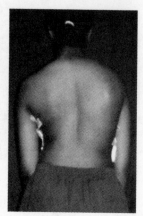

Figure 1   Figure 2   Figure 3

congenital scoliosis are defect of segmentation (*i.e.*, an abnormal separation of the embryo's spinal segments) and defect of formation (*i.e.*, an absence or a lack of a segment of the embryonic spine resulting in deformity). Such malformations of the spine are usually associated with deformities of other organ systems, including the heart, the kidneys, the lungs, and other vital structures. In fact, one study reported that up to sixty percent of all congenital scoliosis cases are related to associated health problems.

Idiopathic scoliosis is different from congenital scoliosis in that it can emerge at any point during a patient's life (except at birth); in fact, the various age ranges during which idiopathic scoliosis may emerge have distinct labels. If idiopathic scoliosis appears in a child any time between infancy and the age of three, it is called infantile scoliosis (fig. 1). While scoliosis, in general, is more prevalent in females than in males, infantile idiopathic scoliosis appears in more boys than girls and commonly manifests itself as a thoracic curve with a left convexity. Interestingly, infantile scoliosis is unlike any other scoliosis in that many cases of infantile scoliosis tend to resolve themselves without medical intervention. Sometimes a very minor scoliotic curve is part of a young child's development and straightens itself out before the child reaches the age of three. This is not to say that infantile idiopathic scoliosis curves should be ignored; if a parent notices a curvature in an infant's spine, he or she should take the infant to a doctor just to make sure that the curve is neither serious nor related to some other problem.

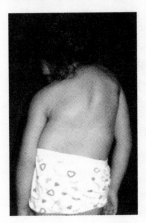

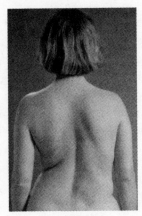

Figure 4

Figure 5

Figure 1: Infantile ideopathic scoliosis in a seven-month-old

Figure 2: Juvenile ideopathic scoliosis in an eight-year-old

Figure 3: Adolescent ideopathic scoliosis

Figure 4: Congenital scoliosis in an eight-year-old

Figure 5: Adult ideopathic scoliosis

If scoliosis appears in a child who is between the ages of four and ten, it is termed juvenile scoliosis (fig. 2). Juvenile idiopathic scoliosis is present in ten to fifteen percent of all idiopathic scoliosis cases. And idiopathic scoliosis in pubescent children of ages ranging from eleven through the teen years is called adolescent idiopathic scoliosis. Adolescent idiopathic scoliosis comprises the vast majority of all idiopathic scoliosis cases. It is likely that most of the cases begin during the juvenile years (ages four to ten); however, they do not often become obvious until a child experiences his or her adolescent growth spurt. Since spinal curves in children increase most when the children are growing, the adolescent growth spurt is the most opportune time for the scoliosis curve to increase dramatically. Hence, teenagers who have just experienced their adolescent growth spurts are often shocked to find that they have developed scoliosis. Interestingly, adolescent idiopathic scoliosis is not random; it tends to follow a series of common patterns. The four most common patterns are thoracic curves, which show a right convexity; thoracolumbar curves, which show a right convexity; lumbar curves, which show a left convexity; and double major curves, consisting of a thoracic curve with a right convexity and a lumbar curve with a left convexity.

In addition to congenital scoliosis (fig. 4), which can be present at birth as a result of vertebral malformation, idiopathic scoliosis affects children (infants and juveniles), teenagers (adolescents), and adults. Adult scoliosis (fig. 5) is most likely to be idiopathic, however; once a person with a naturally straight spine has reached skeletal maturity, he or she might only get scoliosis if there is a likely reason why the scoliosis would emerge. Functional scoliosis in an adult may, of course, appear for any number of reasons (*i.e.,* chronic poor posture) and can be corrected rather easily with postural training. Structural scoliosis in an adult, however, can appear as a consequence of osteoporosis, degenerative arthritis, or any number of other conditions that promote the deterioration of vertebrae.

All forms of scoliosis can occur in any of various areas of the spine. A *thoracic* scoliosis is located in the upper region of the spine, a *thoracolumbar* curve lies in the mid-area of the spine, and a *lumbar* curve is found in the lower spine. A patient may have any one of these three curves, or a combination thereof. For instance, I have what is called a double major curve. My spine resembles a backward letter "S" and is essentially the combination of a right thoracic curve and a left lumbar curve. Some curves may appear to be double major curves, in which both curves are structural, formed independently, and of significant magnitude. Other curves may be a primary curve paired with a compensatory curve of lesser magnitude. In other words, a person may have begun with a right thoracic curve and developed a left lumbar curve later on. The lumbar curve in this case emerged *because of* the thoracic curve; it formed in order to compensate for the patient's primary curve and to maintain a sort of balance in the patient's spine. Certain scoliosis cases exhibit patterns of triple curve deformity, but such cases are extremely rare. Accurate diagnosing of the origin of scoliosis in a patient of any age, along with correctly characterizing the patient's curve, ultimately determines the treatment options.

PROPER DIAGNOSIS

In properly diagnosing scoliosis, it is very important to assess the cause, location, magnitude, and natural history of the deformity. Accurate evaluation and documentation of all aspects of the deformity, including a complete history, a physical examination, and an appropriate X-ray study, are critical components in the process of arriving at a proper diagnosis and treatment. When a doctor examines you for scoliosis, he or she should perform a comprehensive physical examination and conduct a thorough discussion about your medical history, your perception of your

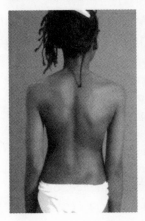 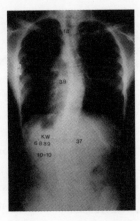

Figure 6: *Adolescent ideopathic double major scoliosis*

Note the patient's back appears straight in the photo, but is obviously curved in the X ray. Because outward signs can be very subtle, regular screening by trained personnel is the most important tool for fighting scoliosis.

health, your preferred activities, and your lifestyle. Only by knowing you, your body, and your scoliosis very well can a doctor recommend the treatment that will be the most beneficial for you. Doctors who fail to perform a comprehensive physical examination risk misdiagnosing you; doctors who are too busy or unconcerned to care about your lifestyle may choose a mode of treatment that, while it may help your scoliosis, may inhibit or upset you. Therefore, in the diagnostic phase, make sure that the doctor is doing all that can be done to properly assess your condition as well as your lifestyle needs.

A doctor cannot properly diagnose a scoliosis deformity by observing the patient alone or by looking at an X ray alone (fig. 6); the physical examination for diagnosing scoliosis includes a number of elements. The spine examination includes evaluation of symmetry in the patient's body; any noticeable asymmetry may be the result of a scoliotic deformity, and the type, severity, and location of the asymmetry provides the doctor with a clue as to the nature of the patient's curve. Typical indications of scoliosis that are visible to the naked eye include an asymmetry of the hips (one is more prominent, or elevated, than the other), a difference in the sizes of the spaces in between the arms and the torso, a crease in either side of waist, an elevation of either shoulder, a prominence of one side of the chest, a protrusion of one shoulder blade, a salient elevation of a particular area of the back (due to an elevation of either the flank area of the back or the rib cage), a discrepancy in leg lengths, and a visibly curved spine. Often, before a person ever reaches an examination room, family members and friends will notice these asymmetries, which may initiate the doctor's visit. In addition to looking at the symmetry of the patient's body, a doctor diagnosing scoliosis may look at the place-

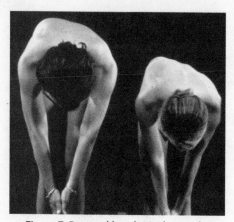

Figure 7: Forward bend. Mother and daughter with similar thoracic curves

ment of the patient's head relative to his or her hips. If a patient's head is directly above his or her hips, this may imply that the patient has maintained some sort of balance (be it because of a very minimal curve or because of a double curve in which one curve appears to balance out the other); if a patient's head is not centered directly above his or her hips, this may imply that the patient has a single, prominent scoliosis curve, or uneven pelvis or leg lengths.

One of the hallmarks of the scoliosis physical examination is the Adams forward bend test, a diagnostic test during which patients stretch their arms out in front of them and slowly bend forward, as if to touch the toes, until their torsos are roughly parallel to the ground. Looking at a patient's back when the patient is in this position, the doctor is able to search for any abnormal elevation of back muscles, rotation of the rib cage, or visible curvature in the spine. Physicians and school nurses usually use the Bunnell scoliometer when performing the Adams forward bend test. The scoliometer is a small plastic apparatus placed at a point on the back (over the spine) and used to detect a discrepancy between elevations of the back. This simple instrument acts as a screen for possible scoliosis, but does not provide the diagnosis of scoliosis. Upon finding a sign of scoliosis, a school nurse or family practitoner may recommend that a child or adult see an orthopedic surgeon. In any case, it is very rare for a patient to end up at the office of an orthopedic surgeon without having first noticed some sort of physical change.

Interestingly, studies have shown that there exists a relationship between scoliometer readings of spine rotation and degree measurements of lateral spine curvature. Thoracic or right convex curves measuring at least twenty-five degrees are apparently associated with scoliometer angles of trunk rotation (ATR) measuring at least nine degrees; lumbar or left convex curves of at least twenty-five degrees are apparently associated with ATR measurements of at least seven degrees. This correlation between trunk rotation measurements and lateral curvature measurements enables pediatricians, school nurses, and scoliosis specialists to predict what the lateral curvature of a patient's spine will be, based on a simple scoliometer reading. For instance, if a child is found to have a trunk rotation of four degrees on a scoliometer, a pediatrician can safely conclude that the lateral curvature of the child's spine is considerably less then twenty-five degrees. The pediatrician can then decide that the child is in need of no treatment other than observation for the time being. This knowledge can reduce the need for unnecessary X rays and follow-up visits to various doctors.

Yet another study directed toward correlating lateral curvature measurements and rotational degree measurements identified a distinct relationship between the two. The authors of this study produced a mathematical formula that they maintain can accurately (with margins of error averaging at about 5.7 degrees) predict the degree of lateral curvature in a patient's spine based on a single scoliometer reading. They hope that, if adopted, this method of correlating the two types of curvature will lessen the cost of school screening programs, decrease the incidence of overdiagnosis (sending children to scoliosis specialists when it is not necessary to do so), and reduce the need for X rays, thereby reducing nonessential exposure to radiation.

As it stands today, radiographs, or X rays, remain a crucial component of diagnosing scoliosis. Depending on the age and situation of the patient, up to four different types of X rays can be taken to diagnose scoliosis. The first and most common type of X ray is the front/back X ray, which gives doctors a front view of the spine. From this X ray, doctors can determine whether the spine is rotated and how much it is laterally curved. In order to accurately measure the degree of curvature shown on the X ray, doctors use the Cobb ruler method to draw what is called a Cobb angle. The first time I saw a doctor draw one on an X ray of mine, I wondered why he was ruining my X ray by writing on it; I soon learned that the degree measurement and the writing is just as important as the X ray itself—it is a documentation of the degree of curvature of your spine at a given point in time. Now, when I look back at old X rays, I appreciate those pencil-written numbers that tell me exactly what degree of curvature I had at any of various points in time when I had X rays taken. The Cobb angle is drawn simply with a pencil and a protractor and tells both the doctor and the patient what the degree of curvature of the spine is. In discussing Cobb angles, I must impart that sometimes even doctors can make mistakes and measure an angle incorrectly. For instance, I was once told by a certain doctor that one of my curves was fifty-three degrees. Several months later, I visited another doctor who told me that the same curve was forty-five degrees. I had stopped growing before either X ray had been taken and had not treated my scoliosis, so I knew that my spine could not have miraculously straightened by itself. I asked the second doctor why there had been a considerable difference between his measurement and the first doctor's measurement, and, upon drawing the Cobb angle once again, this second doctor concluded that inappropriate end points of the vertebrae had been chosen by the first doctor, leading to a falsely high curve magnitude. Thus, I had spent about nine months thinking that my thoracic curve measured fifty-three degrees when it actually measured only forty-five degrees. Aside from egregious errors, doctors are subject to intra- and interobsever error. Any Cobb angle measurement stands the chance of being about three degrees greater than or less than the actual degree of curvature of the spine simply because it is a measurement done by hand and prone to an inevitable, albeit small, margin of human error. So, if a curve has progressed from, say, fifty-two degrees to fifty-four degrees over the course of a year, you need not worry too much; it is likely that the scoliosis has not increased at all. On the other hand, the curve may actually have progressed to fifty-six degrees. As a general rule, then, patients should appreciate and pay great attention to all Cobb angle measurements, yet they should try to take the measurements with awareness that a margin of error does exist.

The standard front/back X ray shows the patient's pelvic bones and spine, and in cases involving growing children, this can be very useful. When diagnosing a growing child with scoliosis and deciding upon a treatment, it is important that a doctor know how close the child is to reaching skeletal maturity. The pelvic X ray that is included in the spinal X ray does the job of illustrating how far along any child or teenager is in his or her growth process. The iliac apophysis bones develop as a child grows; as they develop, they move from the sides of the hip bones to the center of the pelvis, ultimately reaching and fusing with the pelvis once the child has reached skeletal maturity. A patient's Risser sign, formally known as the Risser ossification apophyhsis sign, is a numerical value (for instance, someone may be a "Risser 3") based on the development of this iliac apophysis. The measurement scale, devised by the late Dr. Joseph Risser, measures skeletal maturity on a scale ranging from one to five—one occurring when the child's iliac apophysis bones have not yet formed, and five occurring when the iliac apophysis bones have fused with the pelvis. Yet another X ray that can be used to determine how long a child has left to grow is a hand X ray. An X ray of the patient's hand and wrist is taken and compared to a well-known and widely used medical book of various hand and wrist X rays. This book documents how the development of bones in the hand and wrist relate to skeletal maturity; when a patient's X ray is matched with the book X ray that resembles it most closely, the patient's skeletal maturity may be determined. The hand and wrist X ray and the Risser sign are diagnostic tools used only when diagnosing children and teenagers, for the treatment recommendations for patients of this age will vary according to how far along the patient is in his or her growth process.

A sideview X ray is a third type of X ray used in diagnosing scoliosis. For this X ray, the patient faces sideways, with one of his or her arms essentially "facing" the X ray machine, so that the machine can photograph the spine from the side. This X ray is almost always taken during a standard diagnostic visit to an orthopedic doctor and serves to tell the doctor whether the patient suffers from any abnormal kyphotic (hunchback) or lordotic (swayback) curvature. Every human being is expected to have a small, "normal" amount of both kyphotic and lordotic curvature in his or her spine; too much of either of these types of curvature, however, should be watched and treated just as lateral curvature (scoliosis) is. Sometimes scoliosis is accompanied by an increase or decrease in either the patient's kyphosis or the patient's lordosis; the sideview X ray tells the doctor whether this is the case.

The fourth and final type of X ray that may be used to examine and diagnose a scoliosis curve is known as a bending X ray. The bending X rays (which come in pairs—one for each side that the patient is asked to bend toward) are different from other X rays in that the subject is lying on a table while they are taken. Rather than simply standing in front of an X-ray machine, the patient must be placed beneath one. I remember that, when my first set of bending X rays were taken, I was somewhat intimidated. After I had situated myself on the examination table, one of the nurses asked me to cross my left leg over my right leg, to put my left arm over my head, and to bend as far to the right as I could. I did, and she marveled at how flexible I was.

"Is this too much?" I asked. "Do you want me to go back a little?"

"No, that's good," said the nurse. "Just keep yourself in that position; bend over as far as you can." She left the room while the machine on the ceiling moved over the table and took an X ray of my bent body. Soon the lights turned on, and the nurse reappeared and asked me to do the same thing, but now to the other side.

When I returned to the exam room, the doctor informed my parents and me that the bending X rays were taken to evaluate the flexibility of my spine. He explained that the amount of flexibility in my spine, which happened to be a lot, played a major role in determining how I should be treated. My high level of flexibility showed the doctor that my spine would probably be forced into place quite easily with the help of a back brace; had my spine been more rigid or inflexible, perhaps his treatment suggestion would have been different. Furthermore, the doctor was able to tell from the flexibility I demonstrated in my bending X rays that, if I did eventually need surgery, a greater amount of curve correction could be achieved due to the flexibility of my spine. In fact, the X rays showed that my spine straightened almost completely when I bent to the sides, and this indicated to the doctor that eventual surgery would be likely to leave the treated segment of my spine virtually straight.

Bending X rays, therefore, provide doctors with very important information about how a spine will react to given treatments. These X rays, though not necessary, can be very helpful in diagnosing scoliosis and in finding an appropriate treatment.

When diagnosing patients, doctors should not stop at the physical examination. Taking a patient's history is a crucial part of the diagnostic process. A doctor should ask for a complete medical history, including any past medical problems, any physical symptoms that might be related to the scoliosis, and any other unusual signs or symptoms that the patient has noticed. Doctors may also ask about the patient's family history, for scoliosis is known to be a hereditary disorder, and about the patient's physical interests (*i.e.*, sports, exercises, or other physical activities). These issues are essential in determining whether the scoliosis may be related to any other physical problems and are crucial elements in determining which treatment will best suit the patient.

GENERAL INFORMATION ABOUT SCOLIOSIS
(USEFUL FOR PROPER DIAGNOSIS)

In terms of curve behavior, two different types of scoliosis exist: resolving curves, and progressive curves. Resolving curves either straighten on their own (*i.e.*, as in infantile idiopathic scoliosis cases) or stop progressing at a certain point. Progressive curves, on the other hand, keep progressing until they have been treated effectively. Because there is

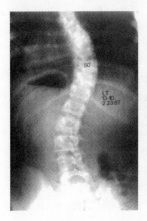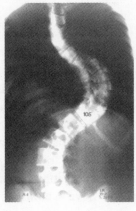

Figure 7: Progressive scoliosis in a teenager. Note rapid progression during the adolescent growth spurt. Bracing attempts to counteract such progression.

such a difference in the behaviors of these two types of curves, the first step in revealing the nature of any scoliosis curve is to determine which type of curve it is. It is by examining specific features on X rays that doctors can differentiate resolving from progressive scoliosis.

Progressive curves are obviously the more serious of the two types of curves because they require constant vigilance on the part of patients and doctors; treatment, be it bracing or surgery; and, sometimes, repeated treatments. Early detection and treatment of progressive curves are absolutely necessary to prevent them from progressing to significant levels. The modes of treatment for progressive scoliosis include body casting (which can eventually be replaced by bracing) in very young patients such as infants; bracing in young children, older children, and teenagers; and eventual surgical stabilization for those whose curves cannot be controlled or maintained with bracing. When a progressive curve reaches a point at which it calls for surgery, the patient has two surgical options: instrumentation without a fusion, or instrumentation plus a fusion of the curve. The surgical recommendation rests upon the treating surgeon and is based on the patient's age, curve flexibility, and curve magnitude. Progressive curves in patients who are nearing or have reached skeletal maturity are usually stabilized with instrumentation (any of various systems of hooks and rods) accompanied by a fusion, in which bone grafts (pieces of bone) are placed in the partially corrected, straighter spine. Patients who are still growing but who are in need of surgery usually receive instrumentation without an accompanying fusion. Surgeons normally use a special sort of instrumentation called subcutaneous rods or subfascials[2] for children who are still growing, so that the children and their spines may continue to grow. Once a child with subcutaneous instrumentation has reached the prepuberty or puberty stage, the implant system will be reinforced with a spine fusion to ensure that the progressive curve will no longer have any chance of progressing.

If a progressive curve is not detected early on, it will continue with its natural history until it inevitably becomes obvious enough to be noticed by someone. The natural history of a scoliosis curve is the history of the curve's progression as dictated by nature; in other words, the *natural history* of a given curve includes what the curve has done in the past and predicts how the curve will act in the future, if left untreated. The natural history of scoliosis—namely, of idiopathic scoliosis—has been studied extensively, and the studies have established that children who are less skeletally mature and have larger curves run the greatest risk of curve progression. Knowledge of the natural history of scoliosis left untreated is normally the basis for a doctor's opinion about the effectiveness of early treatment programs and subsequent recommendations of treatment. Non-scoliosis specialists or doctors who do not have a grasp on scoliosis (its definition, how to diagnose it, and what its natural history is), should not be entrusted with final treatment decisions.

In addition to the studies that have been done on the natural history of scoliosis, there have been extensive studies on the causes of scoliosis. These studies have exposed genetic patterns in the disorder and have consequently led researchers and doctors to conclude that scoliosis is, in fact, a genetic disorder. Like most genetically linked traits, scoliosis has a tendency to act randomly as it passes through generations. On one hand, the disorder may pass over a particular generation of a family or manifest itself in such a minor fashion as to remain unnoticed; on the other hand, it may flourish in a particular family, appearing in and warranting treatment in siblings, parent-child pairs, or grandparent-grandchild pairs.

Specific studies have confirmed hereditary patterns of idiopathic scoliosis in siblings, including twins (both identical and fraternal). Cases in which siblings have in common the trait of scoliosis have been reported in about seven percent of all families with children who have scoliosis. On the intergenerational level, parental scoliosis has been reported in six to fifteen percent of all families with children who have scoliosis. Thus far, genetic research on scoliosis has resulted in an enhanced understanding of where scoliosis comes from and why certain people develop it. Doctors and patients are now looking to genetic research to answer the questions, "Is there any mode of final treatment for scoliosis that is more effective and less difficult than a spine fusion?" and "How can we prevent future generations from having scoliosis?" These frequently asked questions have yet to be answered. While a discrete gene carrying the scoliosis trait and a particular mode of inheritance remain unknown, research teams in various parts of the world are working assiduously each day to find them.

Though idiopathic scoliosis has proven itself to be a hereditary trait, hereditary factors in congenital scoliosis remain rare. The lack of any genetic factor in congenital scoliosis can be attributed to the fact that congenital scoliosis originates because of an abnormal formation of the spine during the period when a human being is an embryo. An anomaly in the vertebral development of an embryo is more likely to be the result of an isolated incident that took place in the mother's womb than the result of a hereditary trait.

Once a patient has been diagnosed with scoliosis and told to resort to a particular treatment, the patient is likely to wonder how his or her spine will behave in the future. The predicted progression of a scoliotic deformity is based on factors including the sex of the patient, the patient's growth potential, (i.e., menarchal status, or Risser sign indicating skeletal growth), and the patient's age at his or her diagnosis. Contrastingly, nonpredictive factors—factors that may or may not have an affect on the patient's lateral scoliosis curve—include a family history of scoliosis, the presence of kyphosis or lordosis, and a rotation of the spine.

As a general rule, a child with a curve measuring nineteen degrees or less and a Risser sign of zero or one has a twenty-two percent risk of progression; yet a child with the same curve who has a Risser sign of two, three, or four has less than a two percent chance of progression. A child with a curve measuring twenty to twenty-nine degrees and a Risser sign of zero or one has a sixty-eight chance of progression, while a child with the same curve and a Risser sign of two, three, or four has only a twenty-two percent risk of progression. Once again, these natural history patterns follow the principle that younger patients with larger curves are at the greatest risk of progression. If scoliosis in an adult or in a child who has reached skeletal maturity continues to progress, it will do so at a rate of one to two degrees per year.

INCIDENCE OF PROGRESSION OF UNTREATED ADOLESCENT IDEOPATHIC SCOLIOSIS WITH THE CROSS CORRELATIONS OF CURVE MAGNITUDE AND RISSER SIGN[3]		
Risser Sign	Magnitude	
	<19 degrees	20–29 degrees
0–1	22%	68%
2–4	1.6%	23%

EARLY DETECTION

Early detection of scoliosis—detection of the curve while it is relatively small—will give way to effective treatment of the curve so that serious physical (health) problems and cosmetic changes can be avoided. While it is impossible to ensure that all scoliosis can be detected early on, it is important to promote as much early detection as possible through the implementation of scoliosis screening by pediatricians and school nurses. In children, it is crucial that the diagnosis be made before or during the growth years, usually when the child is between the ages of ten and fifteen, because a growth period is the time during which scoliosis is likely to progress most rapidly and unexpectedly. If detected before or during a child's major growth spurt, scoliosis may be treated with bracing and its progression effectively halted or slowed, thus preventing the need for surgery in future years. If, however, scoliosis is suddenly noticed in a child or teenager who is no longer a candidate for bracing, the child or teenager may face surgery.

Visual screening for scoliosis is not intended to diagnose the disorder, per se, but rather to detect it. The simple procedure consists of a doctor or school nurse checking for any asymmetry in a child's body, performing the Adams forward bend test, and measuring the spine with a scoliometer to detect any rotation. The Adams forward bend test must not only be performed while the child is facing away from the doctor or nurse, but it must be performed while the doctor or nurse views the child from the side. This sideview is meant to detect any kyphosis (roundback) or lordosis (swayback) that may accompany scoliosis or exist on its own in a given patient.

Since scoliosis is often a painless condition (especially in children and teenagers), it may not come to a nurse's or doctor's attention unless either is looking for it. This is one reason why the principle of scoliosis screening is endorsed by both the Scoliosis Research Society and the American Academy of Orthopedic Surgeons. These and other organizations have long called for routine periodic screening for scoliosis. To date, the American government has mandated school screening in over thirty states across the nation—this statistic being largely due to the work of lobbying parents and patients. The validity of school screening, however, is not felt as strongly by many other nations as it is felt by America. In fact, school screening is an issue that has sparked much debate in the world of scoliosis. Task forces in Britain and Canada, for instance, have done away with school screening programs, deeming them too costly and not very useful. Certain studies have challenged the accuracy of the Adams forward bend test and deemed the incidence of scoliosis in the population too low to warrant potentially costly school screening for everyone. Other studies, however, have concluded that school screening may be conducted in such a way that requires negligible costs. Those who have conducted the pro–school screening studies maintain that the number of scoliosis cases detected via school screening remains high and is instrumental in avoiding countless operative procedures.

SABINA

Sabina's bout with scoliosis began when the nurse at her school was giving the students their annual physical examinations. The fifth graders entered and exited the examination room in an uninterrupted stream until it was Sabina's turn. Having discovered an abnormal curvature in Sabina's spine, the nurse briefly postponed the rest of the students' examinations while she ran downstairs to the kindergarten classroom where Sabina's mother was teaching. She advised Sabina's mother to take Sabina to her pediatrician as soon as possible.

Within hours of the school nurse's discovery, Sabina's mother had taken Sabina to the pediatrician and obtained X rays of her spine. The X rays

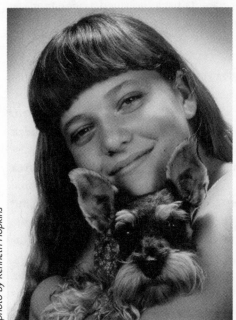

indicated to Sabina's disbelieving mother that her daughter's spine had, in a six-month period, gone from having little or no curvature to having a forty-four degree curve in the thoracic region. While Sabina's mother sat, devastated, gazing at the X-ray films, she heard the pediatrician's voice in the background; he was contacting an orthopedic doctor in Kansas City and arranging an appointment for Sabina.

Just ten days later, the orthopedic doctor in Kansas City told Sabina that she would have to wear a metal

photo by Kenneth Hopkins

back brace for twenty hours each day. Sabina's mother remembers the doctor's gently delivered but hard-hitting ultimatum.

"If you don't follow these directions, you will be crippled by the age of twenty-one. If you do follow the directions, you'll be fine."

"He left us alone," Sabina's mother recalls. "We cried for about forty-five minutes—we just let it all go. But the doctor was really nice. He came back in and said that Sabina was going to be a stronger person for this, which is really true."

For Sabina, the period from January to May of that year was cluttered with more X rays, a lot of measurements, and the psychological obstacles that accompany a scoliosis diagnosis. Sabina dreaded getting the brace and feared looking like something was wrong with her. That May, she and her mother traveled, once again, to Kansas City; the brace was finally ready.

Sabina has now been wearing her back brace faithfully for a few years. The progression of her scoliosis has come to a screeching halt, and her doctor feels that surgery will not be a prospect that Sabina will have to face. Had it not been for the school screening program that caught it, Sabina's scoliosis might have progressed unnoticed for years. Had this been the case, Sabina might not have had the choice to opt for brace treatment; in fact, she probably would have had surgery by this point. Despite any arguments that have been brought forth against school screening, Sabina and her parents have remained, understandably, ardent supporters of the practice.

PEDIATRICIANS WHO LACK UPDATED TREATMENT INFORMATION

Unfortunately, many pediatricians' knowledge of scoliosis is limited. Although pediatricians always know what scoliosis is and how to check patients for scoliosis, they often do not know the complexities of this disorder. While some pediatricians may be very knowledgeable in the area of scoliosis, others may lack the discretion to diagnose a very minimal curve or to suggest an apt treatment for a curve. As a result, children and teenagers are at risk for "slipping through the cracks"—having scoliosis, but being passed over in inadequate diagnostic tests for the disorder. This is not to say that parents and patients should lose trust in pediatricians. Pediatricians are frequently the first doctors to notice scoliosis. However, parents and patients should be aware that not all pediatricians have as keen a familiarity with scoliosis as they should. I know this because I was the victim of one pediatrician's lack of updated treatment information and relatively inappropriate handling of a suggestive scoliometer reading.

BROOKE

"Okay, Brooke, now bend down slowly and try to touch your toes for me," my pediatrician ordered, in his characteristically soft and comforting voice.

I eagerly swung my torso toward my legs, placed my nose between my knees, and laid the palms of my hands on the floor.

"Wow!" the pediatrician exclaimed, laughing, as he did every year. "You sure are flexible aren't you?" A coy smile dashed with a certain childish arrogance flashed across my face, which had taken on a reddish color as blood rushed to my upside-down head.

"Well, it's great that you're so flexible, Brooke, but I need you to come back up a bit and make your torso parallel to the floor," the doctor continued. Satisfied that I had impressed him with my flexibility, I slowly pulled my torso up so that it was perfectly parallel to the floor.

Distracted by the noises outside the examination room, I hadn't noticed that my pediatrician had begun talking to me. Just as I began to pay attention, I heard the words, "I'm just checking to see if your spine is straight."

"Oh, okay," I murmured, distracted again.

After staring at my back from various viewpoints and placing his hands on it in search of any irregularities, my pediatrician laid a small, strange-looking plastic measurement device above the center of my spine. Glancing at the reading on the device, he concluded, "That's great! It's straight as an arrow. Your back is just fine."

This comment yanked me from my childlike daydream. The comment, itself, was in no way captivating; what caught my attention was

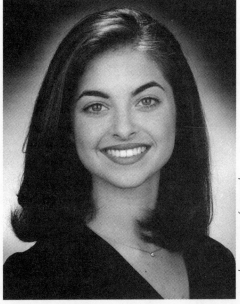

photo by Kenneth Hopkins

that the doctor seemed a bit too surprised about my spine's being straight. The concept that my pediatrician thought my spine might actually have been crooked worried me. After all, I thought that everyone knew that spines are invariably straight; why would my pediatrician have thought otherwise?

"What do you mean?" I asked the doctor, confused. "It isn't possible to have a spine that is not straight, is it?"

"Well, most people have straight spines," he answered, "but there *are* some people whose spines are crooked."

"Whoa, that's so weird," I replied, rather amused by the notion of a crooked spine. My ten-year-old mind then began to conjure up visions of fictional characters, such as the Hunchback of Notre Dame, who had appeared in stories I had read and whose backs were marked by noticeable bending or curvature. Having considerable trouble believing that a real person could actually resemble someone like the Hunchback of Notre Dame, I lost interest in the subject and dismissed it from my mind before I had even left the doctor's office.

Three years and two annual physicals later, I found myself, once again, at my pediatrician's office. As a teenager, I had become bored with the routine physicals that had once fascinated me. I was too old to play with the toys in the waiting room, too "cool" to read the children's books available, and too experienced to wonder what part of my body the doctor would examine next.

After the nurse had checked my weight, height, hearing, sight, cholesterol, and blood pressure, the doctor asked me to bend over and align my torso with the floor so that he could perform the annual spine examination. This year, my desire to show off my flexibility seemed to have waned, so I did not bend over as far or as quickly as I could. I was thirteen now, and old enough to handle the routine physical in what I considered to be a mature fashion. As usual, my doctor laid his hands on my back to search for any asymmetry, viewed my spine from various angles, and placed the now familiar plastic measurement device above my spine.

Soon, enough blood had rushed to my upside-down head to make my face more flushed than rosy. When tears—not tears of emotion, but the type of tears that had blurred my vision each time I had competed with friends to see which of us could maintain a handstand for the longest amount of time—started to fill my eyes, I began to suspect that the spine examination was taking longer that day than it had in previous years. I felt the doctor tip the scoliometer to the left, and then to the right.

I stood inert, still bent in half, while the doctor continued his analysis of my back. Suddenly, a distinct voice cut through the silence. The voice belonged to my mother, who had been sitting in her usual spot—the extra chair in the examining room.

"Is there something wrong?" she asked, rising from her chair.

"Well," the doctor sighed as he, too, rose to an upright position, "Brooke's back is not completely straight." At this, I sprung up and encountered some light-headedness as a result of having shifted positions so quickly. Regaining my composure, I glanced at my mother and sensed that she was panicking.

"What do you mean, 'her back's not straight'?" my mother asked. I grew uneasy. I was annoyed by the prospect of there being something wrong with me; I suddenly wanted to forget about this day, this physical, and this tentative diagnosis.

"Oh my goodness, please don't worry," the pediatrician said, his gentle words and soft smile wrought by an honest concern for my mother's and my mental welfare. "It's not that bad. The curvature I detected is negligible."

"It may be negligible, but it's still there, isn't it?" my mother asked.

"Yes, but I see no need to do anyth—"

"Well, shouldn't we send her to a specialist or something?" my mother argued.

"No," he replied. "Really, I see no need to do anything about this. I've seen curvature in many children's spines during their growth years; normally, their backs straighten out."

"Are you sure we shouldn't take her to some sort of specialist?" my mother asked once again.

"I'm positive," the doctor answered. "All we can do is keep an eye on Brooke's spine. Of course, you *can* take her to another doctor if you want to, but even an orthopedic doctor will tell you that, at this point, there is nothing, other than being vigilant, that you can or should do because she has already begun to menstruate and therefore must be about fully grown."

Before saying goodbye, my doctor imparted a few words of lasting comfort. "Have a great year," he said, "and don't worry about your back. We'll check it again next year just to make sure that it's okay; I'm sure we'll find that it straightened itself right out!" And with that, my mother and I left the office under the impression that my spine was, or would soon be, straight.

In the four years that have passed since that visit to my pediatrician, I have experienced an adolescent growth spurt during which I grew two inches in one year; I discovered my scoliosis long before I was due for another yearly physical at my pediatrician's office; I visited scoliosis specialists and have been shocked to find that what my pediatrician had deemed to be inconsequential scoliosis had progressed to become moderately severe scoliosis during that year of rapid growth; I have been braced for a period of one year and stopped wearing my brace when I reached skeletal maturity; I have accepted that, even though I have stopped growing, my scoliosis has continued to progress; and I have had endless discussions and incessant thoughts about when I should have the surgery that has now become the only treatment option to prevent any further progression.

In retrospect, I regret my doctor's ignorance. Had he known that scoliosis in adolescents progresses most during adolescent growth spurts, he might have been more affirmative when he suggested that I see a scoliosis specialist. Had he known that infantile—and *not* adolescent—scoliosis cases are known to straighten themselves out without the help of treatment, he might not have led me to believe in the virtually impossible notion of my own adolescent scoliosis straightening out. Had he known the basic facts about scoliosis, he might have recommended that I get a brace sooner than I did, thereby giving me ample time to treat my scoliosis. And had he mentioned the word *scoliosis* rather than alluding to some esoteric back problem, my parents and I might have taken his vague warning more seriously or investigated the disorder a bit.

Just a few weeks ago, my nine-year-old sister Chloe visited her pediatrician for her annual physical. Prior to this physical, my mother, who is now very knowledgeable about scoliosis, had noticed a slight elevation in the right thoracic region of Chloe's back. Suspecting that Chloe has scoliosis, for the disorder is hereditary and we already know that it runs in our family, my mother decided to ask the pediatrician about it. The pediatrician utilized the Adams forward bend test and a scoliometer to determine that Chloe does have very minimal scoliosis,[4] but that it is not yet prominent enough to warrant treatment.

"Chloe's curve is very small," the pediatrician said.

"I thought so," my mother agreed. "I just think that we should keep an eye on it, because it could progress at any given moment, and once it reaches about twenty degrees, we'll want to do something about it."

"Twenty degrees!" the pediatrician shrieked. "Isn't that the point at which patients start having surgery for their scoliosis?"

"Are you kidding?" my mother asked, dismayed at the pediatrician's evident ignorance. "Twenty degrees is minimal. Once a child or teenager has a twenty-degree curve, he or she may begin to consider wearing a brace. Surgery doesn't come until much later down the road."

"How do you know all of this?" the pediatrician implored.

"My seventeen-year-old daughter has scoliosis," my mother answered. "Both of her curves are nearing fifty degrees now, and she is deciding when to have her surgery."

"Fifty degrees," the pediatrician echoed. "Wow! That's a big curve."

"Well," my mother said, "it actually isn't. The fifty-degree range *is* the point at which people must consider surgery, but it's nothing devastatingly out of the ordinary. I've heard of many patients whose curves are much worse than Brooke's curves."

"Wow," the pediatrician repeated, apparently unashamed to show her ignorance. "So they use those Harrington rods for the surgeries, now, don't they?"

"No!" my mother exclaimed, now laughing at the pediatrician. "Harrington rods are almost completely obsolete. They were replaced by more modern instrumentation systems years ago."

And so, my mother ended up giving this pediatrician an introductory lesson on scoliosis. Of course, there are many pediatricians who *do* know quite a lot about scoliosis and who can be trusted to give good advice. Pediatricians who are scoliosis-knowledgeable are a great asset to their young patients who may depend solely on their expertise. Parents should not be unreasonably suspicious, but should always be wise and careful when following any doctor's advice.

REACTION TO DIAGNOSIS

An initial scoliosis diagnosis has the power to elicit many reactions from a patient as well as from the patient's parents or spouse. Before concerns about being "different" or having to deal with the scoliosis ever arise, a person who has been diagnosed with the disorder is likely to wrestle with the myriad incipient emotions that speckle the path toward acceptance. These emotional reactions may include shock, disbelief, confusion, guilt, dismay, anger, denial, and sadness, among others.

Some patients struggle with the question, "Why me?" while parents ask themselves, "Is this my fault?" Other patients nod their heads in instant acceptance of their scoliosis, along with whatever treatments it warrants. Some patients like to talk to friends, siblings, parents, doctors, and their fellow patients about scoliosis, gaining support from and finding comfort in each conversation. Others would rather not talk to anyone about their scoliosis, take whatever action is necessary to treat the scoliosis, and put it behind themselves as soon as possible. Whatever the case may be, any reaction to a scoliosis diagnosis is acceptable. As is the case with any disease or disorder, people's reactions to and handlings of scoliosis vary greatly.

I would venture to say that the biggest part of truly accepting one's scoliosis comes from support from family and friends, positive thinking, talking about the problem, letting go of one's emotions, and knowing that one is not alone. If a patient feels alone or isolated, he or she should undoubtedly seek the help of a support group or a friend. The remainder of acceptance comes from putting one's scoliosis into perspective. It may seem like the end of the world is imminent when scoliosis first touches your life, but in reality scoliosis is not the absolute worst thing that can happen to you. It took me a long time to realize this, but when I did, I never looked at having scoliosis the same way again. Of course having scoliosis is nothing to rejoice about, either; it is potentially a very upsetting adversity that must be treated as would any other disappointing reality in life. However, scoliosis patients must remember that they have a disorder which, most likely, can be treated; they have a problem, but it is one that can usually be solved. Though talking to people about your problem, learning more about scoliosis, maintaining an optimistic attitude, being emotionally strong, adhering to treatment, putting your scoliosis into perspective, and trying to live your life as you would if you did not have scoliosis sound like idealistic goals, they are probably the most salutary agents for any scoliosis patient.

My own journey toward acceptance of my scoliosis has taken a very long time. I felt the pang of the initial diagnosis each time I traversed a new threshold of treatment for my scoliosis. The notion of having scoliosis was, at first, almost unreal. When first diagnosed, I was completely shocked and deeply upset. In fact, I was so upset that, after leaving the doctor's office, I rejected the idea of having scoliosis. Internally brooding and occasionally leaking words to my mother, I concluded that this could not be happening to me. I was a *normal* girl; nothing was ever wrong with me. And if anything was ever wrong with my life, *some-one*—usually one of my parents—was bound to be able to fix it for me. This having been the nature of my life for fourteen years, I naturally concluded that my parents would be able to fix this scoliosis problem as well. Surely, other people would have to wear back braces and have surgeries, but not me; I was the invincible Brooke whose life never went awry. I quickly learned that there are some things in life that parents cannot fix, and that no life is without dilemmas.

BROOKE

I was fourteen years old during the summer of 1995, and due to nagging concerns about my back and spine, my mother took me to an orthopedic surgeon. She briefly described our suspicions about my back to the doctor and asked him to take a look at me. He happily agreed, and began to examine my back and spine using the tactics of observation and an Adams forward bend test. He said that although he didn't see anything indicative of a problem, only an X ray would assure him of his assumption. Upon seeing my X ray, the doctor had returned to the examining room where my mother was waiting as I had stood alone in the dark X-ray room. Without warning, he sighed and stated, "God, her scoliosis is pretty bad." My mother was completely unprepared for this news; she fell silent. Of course she was worried, but she, herself, had not seen the X ray and did not have an accurate visual representation to support the doctor's opinion.

"But we're in luck," the doctor continued, "because our spine specialist happens to be here today. I'll have him take a look at the X ray, and we'll be back in a few minutes."

Shortly after he left the examining room, I returned to it. Unaware of the conversation that had just taken place, I nonchalantly took a seat and began to play with my younger sister, who happened to have come with us that day. Then, looking at the model of the human spine and the many posters of spines that decorated the examining room, I began to make jokes about scoliosis. The whole time I was joking, though, I had no idea of how serious my scoliosis might have been. In retrospect, I suppose that I made these jokes in order to lessen the solemnity of the occasion and to make myself feel better. Although I said nothing to my mother at the time, my mind was latent with conflicting ideas. From a logical point of view, I knew that I wouldn't presently be at this doctor's office if there was nothing wrong with my spine. Nevertheless, I couldn't help telling myself, "No, this isn't happening to me. I'm perfectly healthy; nothing's wrong." I denied the possibility of my scoliosis being a problem and told myself that, upon their return, the doctors would tell me that I could go home because everything was all right.

As the doctors entered the examining room, my indifference subsided and was replaced by fear. Emptiness filled my stomach as I waited for someone to speak. Without first talking to my mother about whether or not she wanted me to hear this initial diagnosis, the spine specialist placed my X ray in the viewing box and began explaining it. For a few moments, I heard nothing other than what seemed like a murmuring in the background. Of course the doctor had begun to explain his diagnosis, but all I could concentrate on was that X ray. I sat staring at it, stunned. My mother later told me that when she first looked at the X ray, she was sure that it was a mistake and that it was some other child's X ray. Neither of us had ever actually seen scoliosis before and, up until now, we had been under the natural assumption that my spine was perfectly straight. One can imagine the shock and disbelief we felt when we saw this X ray of a spine literally shaped like a backward letter "S." Not only were we stunned at that, but more at the fact that this was *my* spine. The doctor soon paused and pointed out that the degree measurements of the curves were thirty degrees and thirty-six degrees.

"You're going to need to have surgery for your scoliosis. I don't do this type of surgery, though, so I'll refer you to someone at another hospital who does," he said in an apathetic tone. Once again, denial was my prevailing emotion, but I also felt the beginnings of anger, sadness, and despair. As I looked to my mother for comfort, her eyes met mine, and I knew that we were thinking about the same thing. She was the first to speak.

"Wait a minute," my mother said. "We have to take Brooke's dancing into consideration here."

She proceeded to tell the two doctors in the examining room that I had been dancing since the age of two and that I now danced ballet almost every day. The first realization that I might have to give up my dream began to come into focus as I heard her say to them that I had devoted so much time and effort over the years to improving my technique, practicing various pieces, and performing in shows; and that, in the course of those years, ballet had become my passion.

Now I was shocked into the need to gather information. How would this surgery affect my dancing? How soon after the surgery would I be able to resume dancing? Would I even be able to dance at all? Would I maintain all of my abilities and still be able to perform? The questions were innumerable, and my apprehension was infinite. As if convincing the doctors of my absolute love for dancing would make a difference in their diagnosis, I added to my mother's oration my own feelings about ballet and told the doctors in a very resolute voice that I would *never* think of giving it up.

"Oh, don't worry," one doctor began, trying to reassure me. He said that I would be out of school for a month after the surgery and in a body cast for a few months. As for ballet, I wouldn't be able to dance for a full year following the surgery. The doctor seemed pleased to deliver this information; he sounded as if he thought a year were a short amount of time. In my opinion, though, a year would seem like an eternity without ballet. I later realized how many more questions I would have liked to have asked, but, at the time, I was in too much shock to say much of anything. Shortly after the doctor had briefly explained his diagnosis and suggested treatment, my mother, my sister, and I left the office. Off we went, with my X ray in hand; we were silent, numb, and baffled by the fact that we hadn't noticed my scoliosis before it had gotten so severe.[5] My mother expressed fear, frustration, guilt, and anger. She was very upset by the nonchalance with which the doctor had conveyed this news, and that he had adressed me—at age fourteen years, ten months—without discussing it with her first.

"He could have at least asked me if I wanted you to hear his opinion, before he went ahead and told you that you need surgery!" she exclaimed. "Why haven't we noticed this scoliosis? And, moreover, why didn't your pediatrician warn us about it? He was always so laid back about everything! He should have been more attentive." I silently shrugged in agreement as she picked up the car phone and dialed the number for my father's office.

In comparison with those of my mother, *my* feelings at that point in time seemed negligible. I wasn't exceedingly angry or sad; I simply felt shocked and confused. I suppose that, since this had all happened so quickly, my bewilderment temporarily outweighed my unhappiness. As I sat in the passenger seat, gazing out the window, my mind churned. I thought about going swimming on this hot, sunny day; I dreamed about starting ballet again in the fall; and, every now and then, the prospect of this newfound scoliosis would enter my thoughts, tainting the pretty pictures my mind had created. I heard my mother on the phone with my father, reporting our experience at the orthopedic surgeon's office.

"Don't worry, Brookie," she said, pausing from her conversation with my father. "Dad's going to make some phone calls to other doctors and get their opinions. We're not doing anything until we research this scoliosis a little bit more." She looked at me and said, "Don't worry, sweetie, you're going to be fine. Daddy and I are going to get this all worked out."

But the truth is, there are some things one's parents cannot fix. My scoliosis was (and is) one of them. True, it helped to have parents who wished to be knowledgeable about scoliosis and who were determined to get me the best treatment there is, but the fact still remained that I had scoliosis, and that was not going to change.

After dinner that evening, I started to notice that everyone in my family was being extremely nice to me—unusually nice. My father cleared my place for me just as my mother offered to give me a back rub. My brother, who is two years younger than I am, refrained from provoking our routine sibling rivalry. Instead of being his normal, comedic self and striving to irritate me, he was polite. He was uncharacteristically sincere in asking, "So, how does your back feel, Brooke?" I was touched by my family's sympathy, but I could not help laughing at them.

"You guys, don't worry. There's nothing wrong with me," I said with a smile. "I feel fine. I'm still the same old Brooke that I've always been." They received my carefree confidence with strained smiles.

As I lay in bed that night, I finally began to realize why they had been so sympathetic. With nothing to distract me, I felt the reality of what had been discovered that day finally overcome my confusion and denial. I realized that I had to come to terms with the fact that I had scoliosis. This disorder was now a part of my life, whether I liked it or not, and I had no choice but to acknowledge it and treat it. At that point, I had no idea as to whether or not I needed surgery. I was distraught, and all I could do was ask countless questions. "Why is this happening to *me*? Why didn't I know about it sooner? Do I need to have some horrible, scary surgery? What if I'm never able to dance again?" As the questions multiplied, tears began to roll down my cheeks. They were tears of fear, ignorance, anger, and self-pity. I had no idea what the future held in store, and, therefore, I was afraid. In addition to my fear, I was angry. I was not angry at my parents, my doctors, or myself; I was angry at the world and at life. Until that point in time, nothing had ever been drastically wrong with my life; I had so much to be thankful for and nothing to regret. But now, all of a sudden, I had this deformity called scoliosis, and this scoliosis was going to have an adverse effect on my dancing and on my life. As I continued to analyze my situation, the tears fell faster. I cried myself to sleep.

SEEKING SEVERAL OPINIONS

In attaining a correct diagnosis for scoliosis, it is crucial that a patient seek opinions from various doctors. It is every patient's right to get any number of doctors' opinions. A patient should never follow a single doctor's advice—no matter how reputable the doctor—without first investigating his or her situation through reading, asking questions, and seeing other doctors. Second, third, and sometimes fourth opinions have the potential to offer extra information, different perspectives, and alternate choices.

Sometimes, relutance to seek second opinions is the result of fear. Many people are sensitive to offending their initial doctors. Many times this doctor is the family doctor who has treated the patient for years. The truth is, doctors are rarely offended by the seeking of a second opinion and it is more commonly the rule rather than the exception when dealing with life-altering conditions. Every patient has the right to obtain X rays and medical records, including test results, from any doctor or hospital visited. Do not hesitate to return to a doctor you have already seen, or to ask one doctor for the X rays taken at his or her office if you would like to show those X rays to another doctor. If two doctors' opinions conflict, do not fall into the trap of choosing the opinion that best suits you simply because it is "the easy way out"; seek a third doctor's opinion in order to see which diagnosis or treatment suggestion prevails and which is *really* right for you.

Finally, do not listen to or stay with a doctor whose bedside manner you find unbearable; if a doctor apperars unkind, or uncaring, seek another with whom you aptly relate. You should always be comfortable with your doctor, and your experience with scoliosis, or with any health problem, will be a lot easier if it is handled with the help of a doctor you like and trust.

BROOKE

Two weeks had passed since my initial, dramatic scoliosis diagnosis, and the time had come for my appointment with a recommended scoliosis specialist at the Boston Children's Hospital. My parents and I made a special trip from Connecticut to Boston for the occasion.

In the scoliosis clinic, I found myself surrounded by a sea of children and adolescents holding their back braces. While I was waiting for my name to be called, I noticed a bulletin board covered with letters hanging on the wall. As I began to read the letters, I realized that they had all been written by children and teenagers with scoliosis. They were thank-you letters, written to doctors at the Children's Hospital who had treated or operated on the writers—children with scoliosis. As I read the letters, I was moved by the sincerity with which each of them had been written. Through the accounts of their individual success stories, not only did these patients accomplish the goal of showing their gratitude toward their doctors, but they provided hope for new scoliosis patients such as myself.

The stories of their bravery and optimism immediately mitigated my feelings of fear and anger. For the first time, I read and learned about individuals my age, if not younger, who had undergone spinal fusions for curves of measurements as high as ninety degrees.

"Ninety degrees!" I thought to myself. "Wow! My thirty and thirty-six degree curves will be no problem to take care of." For the first time since my diagnosis, I viewed my curves as being slight, and all of a sudden I felt somewhat lucky.

At the bottom of each letter was a name, an address, and a telephone number. The writers of the letters had kindly included this information along with friendly words such as, "Please call me or write to me if any of you scoliosis patients have questions. I'm willing to share my story and to listen to yours."

What a great idea! I thought. There is no better comfort in a difficult situation than to hear about others who have had to go through the same ordeal. And the people who wrote these letters have actually been through all of it: the pain, the bracing, the surgery, and the recovery. They must know more about dealing with scoliosis than anyone. With a new sense of confidence and a warm feeling inside, I heard the nurse call my name.

Following a history and physical performed by a resident, the specialist came into the room. After perusing the information that had just been recorded by the resident, he began to ask me more questions. He asked if I'd ever had bending films taken, if I was fully grown, and if I'd ever had my hand X ray taken. My answer to all three of these questions was a simple "No."

"Well, then, that's the first thing we need to do," he said. In a moment my parents and I would go to the X-ray department in order to get the necessary films taken, which would determine whether or not I was fully grown. But before we left, the doctor explained to us the ramifications of each possible finding. If I was fully grown at that point, bracing would be out of the question because braces are only effective in patients who are still growing. No surgery would be necessary, however. The doctor said that if I were *his* child, he would not recommend surgery just yet. Instead, he would sit still and simply watch the scoliosis carefully. On the other hand, if I had not finished growing, I would be a candidate for bracing.

Reviewing the X rays quite closely, the doctor and the resident came to the conclusion that I had one and a half years of growth left. The doctor explained to me that because I was in the twenty- to forty-degree range and was still growing, I was a good candidate for a back brace. He continued to explain that if, in the future, surgery became necessary, only my lumbar curve would have to be fused (the thoracic would then naturally compensate and straighten). In this case, I would still maintain most of the flexibility in my back.

"What about dancing?" I asked him, already having explained the importance of ballet in my life. He told me that maintaining most of my flexibility would enable me to dance recreationally throughout my life. However, I would never be able to dance professionally, he informed me, because I still wouldn't have *all* of the back versatility of those with whom I would be competing for a spot in a company.

After having been told that surgery was not necessary right away, I had assumed that my life would not be changed by my scoliosis. I thought that by simply wearing a brace for eighteen hours a day, all of my fears and problems would subside. I was, however, very wrong. Although I only had to wear a brace at this point—which meant that I could continue dancing and performing ballet when I wasn't wearing it—I also had to consider what the future would hold in store for me. I had to face the fact that, one day, I would probably need to have surgery. Would I have the surgery and compromise my love for performing? Or would I continue to perform, allowing my scoliosis to get severe enough to eventually necessitate immediate surgery? Would I even have a choice? Unfortunately, I would not know the answers to these questions until I was actually confronted with surgery as an immediate prospect.

My discussion with the doctor soon came to an end. He had been very careful and exact in his diagnosis, and extremely understanding of the impact scoliosis would have on my lifestyle. Unlike the first doctor I had seen, this doctor took the time to examine every aspect of his patient before voicing his diagnosis. Since my parents and I had traveled out of state to see this doctor, he kindly recommended another doctor in Connecticut we might choose to be my regular doctor.

My parents thought that it would be a good idea to seek a third opinion. A few weeks after our trip to Boston's Children's Hospital, my mother took me to the office of the doctor who had been recommended to us. Upon meeting him, I explained my situation, including the fact that I had heard two different diagnoses by this time.

"Don't tell me what either doctor has said," he told me with a smile. "I'll make *my* diagnosis, and *then* you can compare it to those of the other doctors." And after he had examined both me and my X rays, he said the same thing that the second doctor had said, almost verbatim! While I was not excited about the idea of wearing a brace for eighteen hours each day, I was extremely relieved that I didn't need surgery . . . yet. Toward the end of my visit, this doctor gave us the name of an orthotist I would later visit. The orthotist, he told me, was the person who would make my brace. And so I rested with the prevailing diagnosis and, soon after, obtained a custom-made back brace. Though my encounter with the first doctor I saw was a long time ago, I will forever resent him and the unnecessary angst he put me through; he will always serve as my justification for the advice I give people to get several opinions instead of just one.

INFORMATION INTEGRATION AND TREATMENT DECISIONS

Regardless of how many doctors you see and how much advice you get, the ultimate decision concerning your treatment is up to you, and you alone. Doctors' opinions will vary, statistics and information found in medical books and on the Internet will conflict, and the advice of friends, family, and fellow patients will differ from person to person. Therefore, you are fully responsible for deciding which treatment will be most effective in handling your scoliosis without sacrificing your lifestyle or preferences too much.

Finding a treatment tailored to your scoliosis and your lifestyle has everything to do with seeking information, educating yourself about scoliosis, and taking control of your situation. The process of "taking control" of your scoliosis can entail soliciting a number of doctors' opinions; contacting organizations that can give you advice and send you information; looking up scoliosis in encyclopedias and medical books and on the Internet; trying to learn about the various aspects and implications of scoliosis; examining the treatment options available to you; and asking any questions that may arise in your mind, no matter how foolish or complex they may be. (My personal favorite question to ask doctors is, "What would *you* do if you were in my position?" or, for parents of a child with scoliosis, "What would you do if he/she were *your* child?")

In short, the best thing a scoliosis patient (or the parents of a scoliosis patient) can do is to learn as much as possible about scoliosis in order to gain control of his or her situation. Once a patient has started the process of learning about scoliosis, he or she can speak intelligently to doctors, truly gain understanding of the condition, and make an educated decision about treatment. Try to remain as rational and objective as possible; after all, patients who base their decisions on their preferences alone usually end up hurting themselves and jeopardizing their health in the long run. Similarly, patients who choose to ignore their scoliosis and to remain ignorant and passive in decision making rob themselves of the feeling of control that accompanies the process of demystifying scoliosis.

Be careful though, not to loiter in obtaining treatment for scoliosis. Denise and Erika, a mother and daughter who both have scoliosis, learned this lesson the hard way. When Erika was thirteen years old, her scoliosis, which she had known about since her early childhood, measured fifty degrees in the thoracic region and sixty degrees in the lumbar region. At this point, doctors had told Denise and Erika that Erika was a definite surgical candidate and that she should have surgery as soon as possible. Unsure of whether to trust the opinions of the doctors, Denise took to researching scoliosis. For a year and a half she learned about scoliosis, about surgical methods, and about various doctors and hospitals she was considering for Erika. One and a half years later, when Denise finally felt comfortable in her conclusion to allow Erika to have surgery, she took Erika back to the doctor. Erika, now fourteen and a half years old, had curves measuring sixty degrees in the thoracic region and seventy-four degrees in the lumbar region.

The doctor who had initially told Erika that she needed surgery was now reluctant to perform a spinal fusion on her; Erika's curves had progressed to such high-degree measurements and her spine rotation was so severe that the doctor felt compelled to send her out of state to a special hospital where doctors were willing to handle really difficult cases such as Erika's. This necessitated an out-of-state experience that proved to be quite tumultuous.

Through personal experience, Denise realized that patients should try to learn about scoliosis, but they should limit their pretreatment research to reasonable time frames.

HOW TO BUILD A SUPPORT SYSTEM

It's easy to be overwhelmed by the diagnosis of scoliosis. Concerns about curve progression, the efficacy of bracing, and the possibility of surgery can surely tax the routine coping skills and modes of thinking we use in day-to-day living. What can you do to get your questions answered, keep a positive attitude, and relieve anxiety in between your scheduled doctor visits?

One of the kindest things you can do for yourself when you are first diagnosed is to begin the development of a support system. By a support system I mean other people who have been there, who can talk with you about what is happening now, and tell you what you might expect in the future; people who can listen to you and share their experiences with you; people who have coped with what you are going through, and who can give you their tips, strategies and helpful suggestions; people who can hear you without judging you, and who can empathize with what you might be feeling; and people who can point you toward the information you'll need, so you don't have to go it alone and "reinvent the wheel" by yourself.

Many patients begin their scoliosis treatment by struggling with a maze of information. After developing a support system, many patients have a better capacity for coping, have a different perspective on their treatment options, have a better sense of humor, and feel that their lives are sufficiently enhanced so they can now encourage someone else! Here are some suggestions for developing your support system.

◆ *Start right in your doctor's office.* If you are the diagnosed patient, ask your doctor if you can talk to other patients who have been at your present treatment level. Follow through and connect with them. Indicate who referred you, and ask if they might share their experiences with you. It's also a good idea to speak with someone who has had scoliosis for a while and has adjusted well. Likewise, if you are the parent of a patient, ask your doctor for names of other parents. Connect with them. Find out how they dealt with their situations and what suggestions they might have to offer. This is an important first step in networking.

◆ *Join a local chapter of a national scoliosis support group* (see Resource Directory). Your doctor might direct you there, or you can contact a national organization headquarters to find out the location of the nearest suport group. Many chapters have meetings for teens, apart from older patients and/or parents. Chapters have regular presentations by physicians, surgeons, and other allied health professionals. You'll meet other people in your situation, and you'll be on top of the latest information. You won't feel so alone or overwhelmed.

◆ *Inform yourself.* Find out all you can about scoliosis and its management. Read current books and other publications. The more facts you have, the better prepared you'll be.

◆ *Use the Internet.* Here, you can broaden your information search. You can also use chat rooms, e-mail, medical support bulletin boards, etc., to connect with your peers. This is true for both patients and their parents.

◆ *Tailor your network of support to your individual personality and needs.* As your treatment changes, the type of support you need may also change. Teens may use Internet chat rooms, while parents may need the local support chapter for the face-to-face contact. Both approaches are fine, either alone or together.

◆ *Don't overlook other supporters already around you.* Family, friends, and religious organizations can all be sources of help, advice, and counsel during your scoliosis treatment.

◆ *Talk to a psychologist, social worker, or other mental health professional, perhaps just a few times, or on an ongoing basis.* In this way, you'll get professional input on how to cope with the diagnosis and with feelings and thoughts you may have about your treatment.

Having a good support system can help you to understand that scoliosis is not your whole life, but just a part of it. Your support system can enhance your life, make you feel better about yourself, and put scoliosis in a healthy perspective. A good support system can make your life a whole lot easier!

MARIANNE

"In 1960, a dressmaker discovered my scoliosis. I was twelve years old at the time," Marianne remembers. "She noticed when trying to fit skirts on me that one hip was higher than the other, and she could never get the skirts to fit properly."

This discerning dressmaker suggested that Marianne's mother take her to a doctor to have her back checked. Soon after she had been to the dressmaker, Marianne found herself in an orthopedic doctor's office. X rays were taken, an examination was performed, and the dressmaker's notion that something was wrong with Marianne's back was soon affirmed; the doctor told Marianne that she had scoliosis.

"My only sibling was a Down's Syndrome child, and she was fifteen

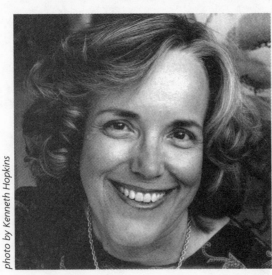

photo by Kenneth Hopkins

months younger than I am, so it was a real blur to my parents to think that now there was something else," Marianne recalls. She remembers having felt bad about having scoliosis and guilty for putting her parents through more unhappiness.

For a couple of years following her initial diagnosis, Marianne had routine six-month checkups with her orthopedist. At each of these checkups, the doctor took more X rays of Marianne's spine—after all, doctors weren't as wary about radiation exposure in 1960 as they are today. In retrospect, Marianne regrets the amount of radiation she underwent as a child and thinks about the health problems it may have caused her.

The orthopedist soon decided that young Marianne's scoliosis was progressing enough to warrant some treatment. He therefore put her into a body cast, hoping to stabilize her curve. In 1960, body casts were still often used as alternatives to back braces, although braces had already been invented at this point.

"They put me in a body cast and cut out slits for my arms," Marianne remembers. "I continued to play sports, and it was very uncomfortable because it would stick to my body and it would hurt. . . . I wore that for six months, and after that, they ordered a Milwaukee brace for me." Soon after the doctor's decision to switch Marianne's treatment from a body cast to a brace, a generically formed and fit Milwaukee brace arrived in Marianne's hometown.

"The brace and a doll were sent to Roanoke, Virginia, where I was being treated; the brace's purpose was to treat my scoliosis, and the doll's purpose was to show me how to put my brace on. The doll had its own miniature brace on."

Thinking that the brace was uncomfortable and that the doll was foolish, thirteen-year-old Marianne quietly accepted her treatment. The 1960s were still days in which people did not challenge the seemingly *divine* advice of medical doctors. And though she was disappointed about having to wear an uncomfortable body cast followed by an equally uncomfortable back brace, Marianne persevered without many complaints.

PAT

"When I was eleven, my mother came in to wash my back when I was in the bathtub, and she noticed that my shoulder blade was protruding," says Pat, sorting through thoughts of children, grandchildren, multiple scoliosis surgeries, and sixty-four years of memories. "She said something about this to my Dad, and he suggested that we speak to my cousin who, coincidentally, had just graduated from medical school." Pat's cousin was very close to her parents, so her parents casually asked him to visit them so that he could look at Pat's back.

"I remember my mother saying to him, 'Ed, something's wrong with

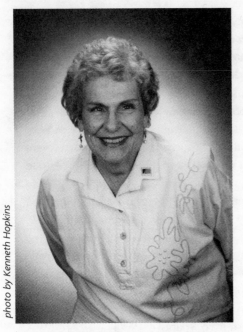

her. This isn't right.' Ed looked at me and agreed with my mother. 'Yes,' he said, 'she does have a problem, and it looks like she has scoliosis.' In the '40s, hardly anyone knew what scoliosis was, but luckily Pat's cousin knew.

Ed set up an appointment for Pat with a scoliosis specialist in Rochester, New York, where Pat had been born. Immediately following her first visit to the doctor, Pat was put into a body cast—"not a brace that could be taken off, but a regular plaster of paris body cast."

This body cast was only the beginning of Pat's lifelong struggle with her scoliosis. Being treated for scoliosis as early as the 1940s, and being a recipient of the rudimentary scoliosis treatments that developed over the years, Pat never benefited from modern surgical instrumentation systems or low-profile back braces. Scoliosis patients in her generation never had the chance to worry about whether wearing a brace or having surgery would threaten their favorite sports or hobbies; they never had to think about their preferences and feelings pertaining to their scoliosis and the treatments they had to undergo. Instead, the scoliosis patients of Pat's era were virtual pioneers who were diagnosed with a very unfamiliar, unheard of disorder and who were primarily concerned with maintaining their health—whether they had to do so by enduring a very rudimentary and painful surgery or by wearing a plaster body cast for months and, sometimes, years.

The courage and commitment involved in accepting scoliosis, adhering to treatment, and making health a primary concern that often characterized young scoliosis patients in the early 1940s are qualities rarely found in young scoliosis patients today. For this reason, I've always found that a wonderful trick to help make brace wearing or surgery easier is to recall what your treatment would have been like fifty years ago, and to be thankful for the comparatively *favorable* treatment options open to you today. Aren't we lucky!

JENNIFER

Jen was diagnosed with scoliosis between 1991 and 1992; she was nine, going on ten, years old at this time. Unlike the majority of scoliosis cases noticed prior to adulthood, Jen's scoliosis was juvenile—and not adolescent—idiopathic scoliosis.

"I noticed it myself," Jen's mother, Jane, remembers. "I just noticed it one day when she was changing and bending over." In addition to her mother spotting a hump in her back, Jen's aunt, who is an X-ray technician, noticed it as well. Jen's aunt told Jane that she should definitely "keep an eye on" Jen's back as she grew.

"As Jen grew, I noticed the change," says Jane. "At one of her physicals, probably the one right before her fourth-grade year in school, I had asked the doctor about Jen's back and told him what I had noticed. At this point, he said, 'I did notice that last year, but I didn't think it was anything to worry about because she still had a lot of growing to do.' " Unfortunately, Jen's pediatrician was terribly mistaken. The time when doctors and parents should worry the *most* about a child's scoliosis curve is when the child has a lot of growing left to do.

Nevertheless Jen's pediatrician did not feel that her curve was severe enough to warrant any sort of treatment at that time. He simply told Jen and her mother to wait for about a year. This suggestion was based on mere assumption; never did the pediatrician suggest that Jen have

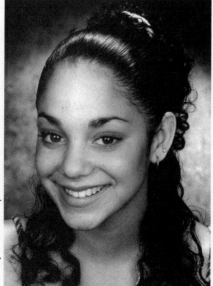

photo by Kenneth Hopkins

an X ray taken to make sure the scoliosis didn't require treatment. He simply told Jen and Jane to do what he *thought* was the right thing to do.

One year later, when Jen was ten years old, the pediatrician noticed that Jen's scoliosis had gotten worse. At this time, he finally sent her to an orthopedic doctor to obtain an X ray. After seeing the X rays, this doctor said to Jen, "Yes, you do have a bit of curvature, but all we have to do right now is keep an eye on it." They took his word, and thanked him for his advice.

"I think that Jen's curve measured about twenty-three degrees when she was just ten years old," Jane says. "We ended up being all confused about numbers because when a second orthopedic doctor got a hold of Jen, he remeasured the X rays. He said that they had been measured incorrectly and that Jen's curves were actually a lot worse than we had thought they were. This doctor still wanted to observe Jen before treating her, and I agreed with him."

Over the course of the next eight months, Jen grew taller, and her mother noticed that her curve was getting worse. She was a very active ten-year-old, dancing jazz and tap, playing softball and basketball, and doing gymnastics all the time. A third orthopedic doctor told the mother and daughter that Jen's curve had progressed from twenty-three degrees to about twenty-eight degrees over the course of the eight months that had passed. He expressed his opinion that Jen "should have been in a brace a year ago."

Feeling as though she and Jen had missed a year and they now had to act quickly, Jane quickly arranged for her daughter to get a brace. She took Jen to visit a fourth orthopedic doctor in order to confirm that bracing was the proper treatment for Jen at this stage. Once the notion was confirmed by this doctor, Jane ordered Jen's back brace.

For several years, Jen was a very loyal brace wearer. Younger children are more likely to do what their parents tell them to do than complain or object; these children are usually very receptive to brace wear. It was not until Jen reached adolescence that she began to have problems with her back brace.

BROOKE

In actuality, I was not diagnosed by my pediatrician or by a school nurse or even by the orthopedic surgeon I first went to see. Interestingly, I was *really* diagnosed by a physiotherapist who was giving me a massage at a hotel in Boston.

Nine months after my August 1994 physical, I had grown almost two inches taller, completed my eighth-grade year in school, celebrated my fourteenth birthday, and gained acceptance to the Boston Ballet School Summer Dance Program. By now, the particular alloy of boldness, autonomy, and apparent invincibility that youth frequently forges had gilded the entirety of my adolescent spirit. My stay in Boston would mark the first time I had lived away from home, and I eagerly awaited its commencement. Once summer had officially begun, I emanated the excitement of knowing that, for the next six weeks, I would have the chance to dance all day, every day.

I led what I considered to be a "normal" life for a fourteen-year-old as I prepared for my stay in Boston, which would begin in late June. I casually went about my daily routine of swimming, sunbathing, sewing ribbons onto pointe shoes, talking on the phone to friends, doing my required summer reading for school, and going out for ice cream. I was so certain, as many teenagers are, that the fundamentally important aspects of my life (*i.e.*, health and general well-being) were so flawless that I didn't even bother to clutter my mind with thoughts about them.

Though the first and second weeks of June took on a fun, carefree quality, they were speckled with bizarre inquiries from my parents and unusual behavior from my clothing and muscles.

"Brooke, I think you're starting to slouch," my mother often said. "What is that posture? Is it a *teenage* thing?"

"Whatever, Mom," I answered, giggling at her silliness. "I'm standing completely straight!"

My mother believed me and admitted that the apparent unevenness she discerned in my posture may have been a mere figment her own eyes had designed. "Oh, it's probably the angle I'm standing at that's making you look like that," she concluded.

As summer continued, temperatures rose, and I replaced my regular warm, layered garments with cool, loose t-shirts. Soon after I had gotten into the habit of wearing baggy shirts, I found that the shirts had an odd tendency to slide towards my left shoulder. At first, I thought nothing of this "shirt sliding"; as if adjusting my shirts were a reflex, I simply pulled the necklines back toward my right shoulder. But eventually the frequency of my having to adjust my shirts and the unfailing tendency of the shirts to slide toward my *left* shoulder in particular led me to the tentative deduction that there may have been a reason why my clothing acted the way it did. Baffled by the question of what the reason behind this mysterious t-shirt behavior was, I blindly concluded that the roots of the enigma lay in my inclination to slouch. I quickly allayed any worries I may have had by promising myself that I would make an honest effort to sit and stand absolutely straight. My solution to the t-shirt problem, however, did not prevent the emergence of other oddities.

One sweltering afternoon, before departing for the pool, I was carefully assessing the appearance of my body in a bathing suit. Being an adolescent girl, I was used to noticing body parts that I was satisfied with as well as those that I wished to change; being a dancer, I was very familiar with each muscle, joint, and tendon in my entire body. For these reasons, I was quite shocked, on this particular day, to discover an aspect of my figure that I had never seen before. While wearing a bikini, I happened to turn sideways so that I could view the right side of my torso; then, I turned the other way so that I could view the left side. Having compared the right and left sides of my body, I became aware of a disparity between the two. While the right side of my waist appeared to have a certain width, the left side appeared to have a notably greater width. Thinking, for a moment, that I was delusional, I looked again at both sides of my waist, and, sure enough, there was a definite difference between the two sides. Captivated by my findings, I began to scrutinize my waist area and soon realized that the discrepancy was not a result of any unevenness in the width of my waist; it was a result of an unevenness in the sizes of my back muscles.

Both amused and annoyed by the small imperfection my body exhibited, I scurried out of my bedroom and fled down the staircase. As I ran, my flip-flops reached each stair before my heels did, creating a symphony of those trademark slapping sounds that only flip-flops can make. Above the racket, I yelled to my father, who was sitting in the family room.

"Hey Dad! Come here and look at my back!"

"What's the matter with your back?" he asked.

"Look!" I exclaimed, turning around so that he could see my back muscles, "One side's bigger than the other!"

"Oh. Your left lower back muscle is just more developed than your right," he said. "It's probably due to something you've been doing in ballet class; it's nothing to worry about."

"Yeah, I guess that could be it," I agreed. "I mean, my legs are pretty muscular from dancing, so why wouldn't my back be?"

"Right."

"But I still don't like the way it looks," I complained. "I look lopsided or something."

"Don't worry about it!" my father said. "If you really want to fix it, just try to build up your right lower back muscle. But, honestly, it's hardly noticeable."

I trusted my father's words and conceded that the difference in the sizes of my back muscles was only obvious to those who observed my back with scrutiny. Most people weren't bound to notice the discrepancy. Furthermore, anyone who did notice the discrepancy would attribute it to my being a dancer, whose body was muscular in general. With that in mind, I declared to my family that I was ready to go to the pool.

As I passed by my mother on the way to the car, I heard her say, "Wow! You look great in that bathing suit, honey!"

"Thanks, Mom!" I replied as I sauntered to the car, newly confident about my handsomely unique musculature.

Later that summer, I was living in one of the dormitories at a college in Boston with all of the other students from the Boston Ballet School Summer Dance Program. Since I was busy learning different dancing techniques, attending a multitude of dance classes each day, meeting new friends from all over the country, and getting to know my way around the city, I hardly noticed that the muscles—especially the overdeveloped lower left muscle—in my back had begun to ache almost chronically.

Toward the end of the long walk from the dormitory to the dance studio every morning, I would feel a throbbing pain in my back. I chose to ignore this aching, telling myself that I would stretch out my back when I arrived at the studio, and forged ahead, not wanting to be late for my morning ballet class. Long walks, though, were not the only occasions on which my back would hurt. There were times in ballet classes, for instance, when I would strain myself to heighten my arabesque and feel sudden pangs of pain in my back. Unwilling to lower my leg or to stop dancing for the moment (because that type of behavior would have been considered poor ballet class etiquette), I chose to endure the pain until the music had ended. Then, I would casually dangle my torso in the direction of the floor until I felt some sort of stretch in the muscles that were in spasms. Redirecting my attention to the teachers, who were usually demonstrating the next exercise, I soon forgot about the pain in my back.

Although I was savoring my first taste of freedom in Boston, I was always amenable to my parents' coming to visit me on weekends, when I didn't have any dance classes or seminars to attend. One Saturday, my parents came to Boston, and we spent the day walking, shopping, and eating lunch in the city. It was during the latter half of that afternoon that we decided to return to my parents' hotel and visit the pool and health club. Though I hadn't mentioned it to either of my parents, my back was aching from all of the walking, and I looked forward to a cool, relaxing swim in the pool.

As I sat on the edge of the pool, dipping my legs into the water, my mother suggested a swim.

"A swim sounds like a good idea to me," I said. "Maybe it will make my back feel better."

"What's the matter with your back?"

"Oh, nothing. My muscles are just aching, that's all."

"Why don't you get a massage? That will make you feel a lot better," my mother suggested.

"My back is fine; it's really not a big deal," I said. But my parents persisted, and my father made an appointment that same day for a massage.

As I opened the door of the massage room, I encountered a woman dressed in hotel staff clothing. She looked at me and asked, "Are you here for a massage?"

"Yes," I answered. "Are you the masseuse?"

"Well, actually I'm a physiotherapist, but I do the massages here."

"Oh, okay," I said, smiling innocently and having absolutely no idea what a physiotherapist was.

I walked into the nearby massage room—a quiet little room filled with dim lighting, relaxing music, and an aromatherapeutic scent. I had just lain on the massage table and covered myself with towels when I heard a barely audible knock on the door.

The door slid open, and the physiotherapist walked into the room, closing the door behind her. She was a soft-spoken woman, probably in her thirties, with a friendly demeanor and an obscure eastern European accent.

"Is there any particular part of your body that is hurting you?" she asked before she began.

"Well, my back has been hurting me a little, but all of my muscles are tired and achy because I've been involved in a lot of physical activity this summer."

"Okay," she said as she began the massage. Though she was a stranger, her bearing was almost maternal. Her unfamiliar hands worked with a certain combination of professional adeptness and polite distance that made me perfectly comfortable during the massage; her periodic explanations of which muscles she was focusing on and why she was focusing on them made me feel certain that she knew what she was doing; and her unobtrusively convivial discussion made me feel as though I had known her for a long time.

Utterly relaxed and enjoying my massage, I asked the woman, "So what, exactly, is a physiotherapist?"

"Oh," she said, smiling. She seemed to be amused by my interest in her profession. "Well, a physiotherapist knows a bit more about the body and the way it works than a regular masseuse does. A physiotherapist actually goes to school to learn about the parts and mechanics of the human body."

As the massage continued, I closed my eyes and lost myself in the repetitions of the relaxation music. Eventually the physiotherapist's voice gently pulled me from my light quasislumber.

"Can you please turn over now?" she asked.

"Sure, no problem," I mumbled, turning my body over so that I was lying face down.

Soon, the woman's hands reached my back. I wondered what she would say about my back muscles. I could almost hear her exclaiming, "Wow! This muscle really *is* in spasm, isn't it?" or, "You have a big knot in this muscle, but don't worry, I'll massage it out." Suddenly, my thoughts were interrupted by her voice.

"Hey, you didn't tell me that you have scoliosis!" she exclaimed. "No wonder your back muscles are hurting you. The scoliosis looks like it may be serious. Do you know what your degrees of curvature are?"

Whenever I tell people this story, they ask if I was scared or upset when the physiotherapist brought this shocking news to light. My response is that I was not frightened, sad, or concerned when I heard the physiotherapist's words. One might wonder why I had no emotional response to this potentially shocking and dramatic (though unofficial) diagnosis; the reason is simply that I had absolutely no idea what the woman was talking about.

"What did you say? Scoli . . . what?" I asked, entirely confused by the woman's remark.

"Scol*iosis*," she said. "You know, a curvature of the spine."

"Oh my goodness! You mean that my spine isn't straight?"

"No, it's not straight. You have scoliosis." She paused. "Are you telling me that no one has ever told you this before?"

"Well, my pediatrician mentioned something about my spine not being straight, but that was last year," I replied. "Besides, he said that it would straighten out—but I guess it didn't! That's so funny!" Knowing nothing about scoliosis or its implications and treatments, I took the news about my spine rather lightly. In fact, I was amused by the correlation between what my pediatrician had said a year before and what the physiotherapist was saying now.

"You must tell your parents about this," the woman continued, with a note of casual concern in her voice. "They should take you to see a doctor who will check your back."

"Okay," I said, obediently. Still, I had no clear understanding of this so-called scoliosis that the physiotherapist was talking about. I would mention it to my parents, but I thought nothing of it. My mindset remained serenely nonchalant as the woman completed my massage.

As I shed my towels and put on my clothes, I mulled over what the physiotherapist had said. Still indifferent to my newfound scoliosis, I walked out of the massage room and exited the women's locker room. When I opened the locker room door, I immediately saw that my mother, my father, and the physiotherapist had formed a triangle of discussion by the pool. I walked in their direction and, upon reaching them, announced my presence with a simple "Hello."

My parents seemed shocked by what the woman was telling them. Because my father is a doctor and my mother is a nurse, they were baffled by the fact that they, themselves, hadn't realized that there was something wrong with my back. Thus, they were too busy listening to the words of the physiotherapist to respond to my greeting. She had told my parents that, since my spine was considerably curved, my back muscles had to compensate in order for me to stand up straight. This job of compensation required my muscles to be overworked, which is why they often had spasms. The physiotherapist did not know exactly how serious my scoliosis was, but she thought that getting an X ray would be worth my while.

My parents and I were somewhat concerned, though in no way alarmed by the news of my scoliosis. In retrospect, I see that our equanimity in this situation was a direct result of our ignorance about scoliosis. Not one of us—my mother, my father, or I—had any idea that my scoliosis could or would have any sort of impact on my health or on my life.

CHAPTER 2

Bracing: The Conservative Treatment Option

Somewhere between observing a scoliosis deformity and surgically correcting it lies an intermediate treatment known simply as "bracing." The broad term, bracing, indicates the wearing of either a removable back brace or a permanent body cast by a person who has scoliosis. Back braces are composed primarily of molded plastic (though some have metal components); are manufactured in a variety of shapes, sizes, and models; and may span any area from the hip bones to the chin. Body casts are made of plaster of paris and are only used for very young children exhibiting notable scoliosis; as these children mature, their body casts are replaced by back braces.

Scoliosis patients who wish to treat their scoliosis but would rather not have surgery often prefer bracing as a treatment option because it is more proactive than observation, yet more conservative than surgery. Regardless of how much someone would *prefer* bracing over other treatments, though, not everyone is an appropriate candidate for brace wear. Be aware that bracing has varying effects on the wearer. Determining a candidate's viability for bracing involves a careful evaluation—for both the doctor and the patient—of factors including age, skeletal maturity, curve magnitude, history of scoliosis, and inclination toward compliance with a prescribed bracing plan.

HOW AND WHY DOES BRACING WORK?

Within the molded plastic bodice of a back brace are foamy pads. These pads, which vary in shape and size, are placed strategically so that they touch and push on the back in areas physically affected by your unique curve. For instance, if you have a right thoracic curve and a prominent muscle or rib hump in the upper right region of your back, your brace will most likely have a pad placed in its upper right region. This pad will push against your protruding back, and thus against the rib leading to the apex of your right thoracic curve, providing enough force to counteract your spine's natural tendency to curve in that direction. If you have a very high thoracic curve, you may have a brace with a neck ring and chin piece. These mechanisms pull up your neck and chin, forcing them to be (comfortably) straight and forbidding them from sinking into the curvature that rests in your spine.

By way of tight-fitting foam pads and supportive, metal components such as neck rings, back braces force your spine into a temporarily straight position. Once you have been wearing your brace for several hours or days, X rays taken while wearing the brace will confirm that your spine has been forced into a considerably straighter position. A common misconception is that back braces are intended to correct preexisting curves. The truth is that *back braces are neither able nor meant to correct preexisting curves.* This is apparent in the fact that once you have had your brace off for several hours, X rays taken with the brace off will show that your spine has returned to its natural, curved position. Knowing that back braces do not result in instant, dramatic, permanent correction of scoliosis may lead you to doubt that bracing is a justifiable treatment, but innumerable studies show that brace wear, when it is practiced continuously by someone who is still growing, is a very effective means of controlling scoliosis in the majority of cases.

If you are a child or adolescent who is still growing, continued wear of a back brace can actually deter your spine from taking its natural, curved path as it grows. Children and adolescents who wear back braces find that once they reach skeletal maturity, their spines are not as curved as they would have been had they not worn their back braces. Success with bracing when applied to growing spines is attributed to the fact that growing spines are flexible and manipulatable; when they are continually forced into a straight position, they tend to adhere to that straight path as they grow.

Mature spines, unlike growing spines, tend to be quite stubborn. Bracing in adolescents who have already reached skeletal maturity will not result in a slowing or halting of the scoliosis. If you are a "grown" teenager or adult, wearing a back brace may temporarily "correct" your scoliosis—perhaps alleviating some of your back pain in the process—for the time during which the brace is on your body. Once the brace is removed, however, your spine will return to its naturally curved position. If you are fully grown, your spine has hardened; the time to influence its growth pattern has passed.

HOW DO DOCTORS DECIDE WHO IS A CANDIDATE FOR BRACING?

It is customary for a doctor to perform a complete examination of you before recommending any treatment modality. A thorough examination for scoliosis includes the Adams forward bend test (described in chapter 1), observation of your body while you are standing erect to check for any asymmetry, assessment of your legs to check for apparent or actual discrepancies in their lengths, and a discussion about your physicality, any difficulties you may have with activities, and any known history of scoliosis in your family.

A physical examination is important because it discloses the nature of your curve and lets your doctor know whether it is a curve that will respond well to bracing. Curves that will respond well to bracing normally include curves measuring between twenty and forty degrees in patients who are still actively growing. A discussion about your lifestyle and your attitude toward bracing is important, as well, because it informs the doctor as to whether your life and attitude will permit brace wear. If you will not wear a brace to work or to school, or if you are an athlete who practices a sport for six hours each day, you may never wear your back brace for the prescribed amount of time. Factors such as this play a large role in a doctor's decision whether to brace you.

For both children and adults, the decision of whether or not to try bracing is a relatively simple one. As a general rule, doctors prescribe braces for children (ages three to ten) and growing adolescents whose curves measure between twenty and forty degrees. Since children are still growing, their spines are still malleable; and since curves ranging from twenty to forty degrees are moderate, they are relatively controllable by brace wear. Doctors rarely prescribe braces for adults (age eighteen and up) because all adults have reached skeletal maturity, and braces will have no effect on their scoliosis curves. For teenagers, however, the question of whether or not to try bracing is a difficult one for both the patient and the doctor to answer.

Teenagehood, or adolescence, is the infamous "gray area" of bracing because it is during adolescence that people start the race toward skeletal maturity. Prior to your adolescent growth spurt, you have a lot of time left to grow—a lot of time in which a brace could have an effect on your spine; after your growth spurt, your time for growing—and for bracing—has run out. Determining whether or not you are a candidate for bracing, therefore, has to do not only with your curve magnitude, but with the amount of growing you have done. A doctor's examination of an adolescent is more involved than an examination of a child or an adult. A thorough examination will include a number of tests and tactics that determine not only exactly how much growing you have left to do, but also how much time that growing will take.

An examination of an adolescent scoliosis patient includes questions about the onset of menarche and development of breasts and axillary (underarm) hair in female patients; questions about the appearance of facial and axillary hair in male patients; and questions about the beginning of the adolescent growth spurt and an assessment of peak height velocity (when the patient's growth reaches its fastest pace) as well as observation of X rays of the pelvic region (to determine the Risser sign) or of the hand and wrist in order to estimate how much "growing time" is left, in both male and female patients. I used to think it strange when doctors asked me when I had gotten my first period or when I *thought* I had begun my adolescent growth spurt. I was embarrassed by some of the doctors' questions and humored by others. I could not figure out why many of the questions I was asked were relevant. I now understand the complexity of treatment decision making and the myriad of factors involved.

AGE, GROWTH, AND SKELETAL MATURITY

Due to the impressionability of growing spines as compared to the obstinacy of hard, set, mature spines, back braces and body casts designed to slow or halt the progression of scoliosis are only effective in patients who are still growing. Also, due to the relatively pliable nature of growing spines is the fact that scoliosis increases most rapidly during skeletal growth (*i.e.*, throughout childhood and especially during the adolescent growth spurt). To determine whether someone is a candidate for effective brace wear, therefore, doctors must first determine the amount of time for which that person will continue to grow—in other words, how far the person is from reaching skeletal maturity.

Naturally, children are far from reaching skeletal maturity; thus, if their scoliosis call for nonoperative treatment, they are immediately braced. Adolescents may or may not have a substantial amount of growth remaining; a given adolescent may have anywhere from a few years to a few months of growth left when diagnosed with scoliosis. It is of the utmost importance to determine an adolescent scoliosis patient's proximity to skeletal maturity before bracing him or her.

When it comes to determining skeletal maturity, a major point of confusion lies in the difference between your chronological age and your skeletal (biological) age. Your chronological age is your age in years; your skeletal (biological) age—which may or may not advance at the same pace as your chronological age—is the apparent age of your body and development of the skeletal system, including the spinal column. There can be a discrepancy between chronological age and biological age. Skeletal maturity does not necessarily reflect how old you are; it merely indicates the apparent development of your bones. I am a typical example of someone whose chronological age and biological age differed. I was diagnosed with scoliosis when I was fourteen years and ten months old. Although I was technically about fifteen years old at the time, X rays showed that my bone growth resembled that of the average thirteen-and-a-half year old. In other words, I was a year and a half "behind" in my growing. This news was well received because it meant that, although most people my age were nearing the ends of their growth periods, I still had one and a half years of growth remaining. Because I had that much time left to grow and because my curves were in the thirty-degree range at the time, I was considered a candidate for bracing.

THE IMPORTANCE OF CURVE MAGNITUDE

The magnitude of the spinal curve is a factor that is equally as significant as skeletal maturity when determining viability for bracing. Opinions concerning the relationship between curve magnitude and "braceability" will inevitably vary from doctor to doctor, but the following reckonings are generally accepted.

Periodic observation by your doctor is the preferred treatment for all curves measuring less than twenty degrees. If your curve demonstrates progression[6] past twenty-five degrees, and if you are still growing, most doctors will recommend brace treatment on a full-time basis. If you are still growing and have a curve that measures thirty to thirty-nine degrees upon diagnosis, you are likely to be recommended for bracing at this initial doctor's visit. In this case, though your doctor has not documented any progression of your curve, he or she can safely assume that a curve of magnitude thirty degrees or more will progress and require treatment.

If you have a Risser sign of 0 or 1, are premenarchal (if female), and have a twenty- to twenty-nine-degree curve that has demonstrated progression, bracing is the right treatment for you. In the same situation, if you have a Risser sign of 4 or 5, bracing will not have much of an effect on your curve. If you have a Risser sign of 2, 3, or 4 and a curve measuring twenty to twenty nine degrees, your doctor will most likely wait until your curve progresses six or more degrees before bracing will be recommended. In general, physicians tend to reserve brace treatment for curves greater than twenty-five degrees that have demonstrated progression, as well as for curves in the thirty- and forty-degree ranges, whose measurements alone are proof enough that they will progress.

Just as some curves are too insignificant to warrant brace treatment, certain curves are just too severe and too progressive to be treated effectively by brace wear; progressive curves exceeding fifty to sixty degrees despite use of an adequate back brace will inevitably require surgical treatment.

CURVE MAGNITUDE + GROWTH STATUS = TREATMENT DECISION[6]

Curve Magnitude	Active Growth	No Active Growth
0–19 degrees	Observation	Observation, discharge
20–29 degrees	Observation or Bracing	Observation
30–39 degrees	Bracing	Observation
>40 degrees	Surgery	Observation or Surgery

THE BEHAVIOR AND PROGRESSION OF SCOLIOSIS

If you are a child or teenager, you are probably still growing, and your curve is bound to progress as you continue to grow. Once you have stopped growing, your curve can do either one of two things; it can stop progressing and stabilize in its position, or it can continue to progress. Regardless of the measures you take to treat your scoliosis, anything can happen once you have stopped growing. You are in luck if you find that your curve is not progressing; in such a case, you will seldom have to worry about your scoliosis again. However, you are in good company if you find that your curve is continuing to progress after you have reached skeletal maturity.

There are several reasons why curves may progress even after the spine has stopped growing. One is that the muscles in your back have already developed in certain ways as a result of your scoliosis and will pull your spine further into the curved position it knows so well; another is simply that natural forces such as gravity will pull your spine further down into its curved position; and a final reason (for older adults) is that aging may lead to a slight deterioration of your bones and produce in your spine a tendency to curve.

If surgery is not indicated once you reach skeletal maturity, the only thing to do is wait and see if your curve continues to progress. If, through your physician's observation and periodic X rays, you find that your curve is still progressing, know that during your biological/skeletal adult life (which may begin between the ages of sixteen and twenty years old) scoliosis curves progress an average of one degree per year, until surgery eventually becomes necessary. Knowing this, you may be able to gauge how curved your spine will be in ten, fifteen, or twenty years, providing a logical and realistic framework for the decision about the best time to have surgery.

WHEN IS A BACK BRACE RECOMMENDED FOR AN ADULT?

Occasionally, back braces are used by adult scoliosis patients who are not surgical candidates as a means of warding off back pain and temporarily straightening posture. If you are an adult whose scoliosis is the cause of back pain or postural difficulty, and if you have either elected not to have surgery or been told that you are not a candidate for surgery, you may prefer to wear a back brace.

A certain percentage of older adult patients for whom surgery is not recommended (because of osteoporosis, arthritis, and other health reasons)
resort to bracing. Additionally, younger adults whose scoliosis curves are
not so severe as to necessitate surgery sometimes turn to back braces for
the temporary straightening of poor posture and the relief of muscle pain.

ARE THERE ANY RISKS INVOLVED IN BRACING?

Studies show that a back brace can decrease your pulmonary function
(breathing ability) while you are in the brace and immediately after
removal. This is because back braces can sometimes be so tight that they
squeeze your body, leaving little room for your lungs to expand. But this
is common knowledge; anyone who has ever tried to climb a flight of
stairs or to go for a walk or run while wearing a back brace can tell you
this. Brace wearers are bound to experience shortness of breath at times,
and learning to take mostly little breaths and to breathe slowly and
deeply every now and then is a large part of getting used to a back brace.
If, at any moment, it becomes *very* difficult to breathe, do not be afraid
to quickly take your brace off while you catch your breath.

While breathing restrictions created by back braces are a point of concern for some people (especially those who have asthma), the studies
showing the effects of back braces on pulmonary function do mention
that once you have stopped wearing your brace, or even if you have taken
it off for a few hours, your breathing ability should return to normal.

Interestingly, in some cases, people claim that bracing has actually
helped their pulmonary function. If you have a considerable amount of
spinal rotation, your ribs, which are rotated as well, may be pressing on
your lungs and making it slightly difficult for you to breathe. A brace,
which temporarily straightens your spine, may decrease the rotation of
the spine and, therefore, decrease the rib-related pressure on your lungs,
making it easier for you to breathe.

Another concern related to bracing is the effect of back braces on a
growing patient's bone density. The concept of bracing, for some, may
evoke visions of bodies being mercilessly bound and of tight-fitting
braces thwarting the normal development of bones in the spine and
hips. If you are a brace-wearer, you need not worry; these types of
visions are, in reality, unfounded and false. Studies show that continued
brace wear in adolescent scoliosis patients does not adversely effect
bone density or the normal development of spine and hip bones.

BRACE TYPES AND THEIR PURPOSES

Back braces exist in a variety of models, shapes, sizes, and colors; therefore, while all braces are essentially alike, no two are exactly the same. Regardless of their categorizations, all scoliosis back braces share a common purpose. They are meant to improve scoliosis-related deformity (*i.e.*, rib humps and overdeveloped back muscles), to prevent curve progression for an extended period of time until you have reached skeletal maturity, and to provide you with postural comfort and stability. While braces cannot correct scoliotic curves, they can delay or stop the progression of the curves, thereby providing their wearers with a realistic hope of avoiding surgery in the long run.

There are four general categories of scoliosis braces known as the *CTLSO*—cervical thoracolumbar sacral orthosis (figs. 1–2), the *TLSO*—thoracolumbosacral orthosis (figs. 3–4), the *LSO*—lumbosacral orthosis (fig. 5), and the *bending* brace. These complex brace names are frequently used among doctors but are rarely used among patients. You are likely to hear of the simpler names that have been assigned to the various kinds of braces; these more common names come from the brace's city of origin and include the *Milwaukee* (CTLSO) brace, the *Boston* (TLSO and LSO) brace, and the *Charleston* (bending) brace. In addition to these braces, various models of braces that follow the Boston brace prototype have been developed over the years. These braces are distinguished from one another by subtle nuances in their styles; however, they are all quite similar and are sometimes characterized, simply, as Boston braces. The brace models that fall under the classification known as Boston braces include the Pasadena, the Wilmington, and the Miami; their European counterparts are the Riviera, the Ponte, and the Lyon.

Once your doctor has determined that you are a candidate for bracing, the decision of which brace model will best suit your particular scoliosis curve must be made. No one model is incontrovertibly "better" than another with respect to effectiveness; the success of any brace is a direct result of both how well the brace fits your curve and how loyal you are to wearing your brace. Each model has a distinct style that caters to the specific needs of patients for whom that particular model is recommended. Individual doctors also tend to have individual preferences when it comes to choosing a brace model; often, the only real difference between two models is just that—personal preference.

The Milwaukee brace was introduced in 1946 by two physicians

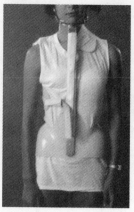
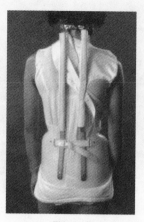
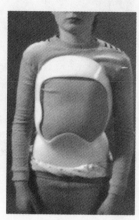

Figure 1   *Figure 2*   *Figure 3*

named Blount and Schmidt. The brace had originally been crafted for the purpose of supporting patients postoperatively; however, doctors soon discovered that it was even more useful and effective in patients who had not yet undergone surgery for their scoliosis. And so the beginning of nonoperative treatment for scoliosis arrived with the dawn of the Milwaukee brace, which patients are asked to wear for up to twenty-three hours each day. This type of brace is usually indicated for patients who have thoracic curves (curves in the upper region of the back) with apexes at or above the T7 vertebra, or patients who have double major curves. Founded on the idea of traction, the brace consists of a molded plastic pelvic section that is normally custom fit to match the patient's figure. Narrow steel rods—one in the front, and two in the back—run from the brace's plastic pelvic section to a ring encircling the patient's neck. Pads are placed within the brace to apply force to certain areas of the back (these areas vary according to the patient and his or her unique scoliosis curve) in order to provide curve correction while the patient is actively wearing the brace. The Milwaukee brace is also often characterized by a chin piece on which the patient can rest his or her head. Though the extension of the Milwaukee brace up to the neck is thought, by many, to be both uncomfortable and unfavorable, it is the distinguishing feature that enables the brace to be effective in treating those "higher" (closer to the neck than to the sacrum) curves.

The Boston brace is normally used for patients who have lumbar (in the lower region of the back)[8] or thoracolumbar (in the middle region of the back) curves. In more technical terms, the group of braces bearing the general name "Boston" is usually suitable for curves with apexes at or

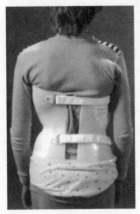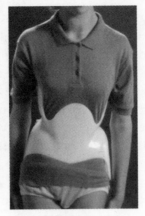

Figure 1: CTLSO—Milwaukee Brace, front view

Figure 2: CTLSO—Back view

Figure 3: TLSO—Low-profile Boston brace for thoracic scoliosis, front view

Figure 4: TLSO—Back view

Figure 5: LSO—Low-profile Boston brace for lumbar scoliosis, front view

Figure 4 Figure 5

below the T7 vertabrae. As in the Milwaukee brace, various pads (and, sometimes, extensions such as underarm slings as well) are placed in the Boston brace to provide specific forces to effectively maintain the patient's scoliosis curve in the corrected position during the time that the patient is in the brace. And, like the Milwaukee brace, the Boston brace is usually worn by patients for anywhere from eighteen to twenty-three hours each day. There are two main varieties of the Boston brace: the TLSO and the LSO. Though the two types of Boston braces are essentially the same, the TLSO extends up to one or both underarms while the LSO extends only to the lower thoracic region of the patient's back. The factor that may determine whether a patient wears the TLSO or the LSO is the location of the patient's curve. Curves that are in the upper lumbar (verging on the thoracolumbar) region, or lumbar curves accompanied by minor thoracic curves will be braces with the torso-spanning TLSO. And curves that are strictly in the lower lumbar region and show little or no thoracic component (*i.e.*, a compensatory curve) will be braced with an LSO. Cosmetically, the "low-profile" Boston brace is usually preferred to the Milwaukee brace because the Boston brace may be fully covered by clothing, whereas the neck ring on the Milwaukee brace is difficult to conceal.

The Charleston nighttime bending brace is different from both the Milwaukee and Boston braces in that it is only worn at night. The Charleston is a plastic brace, otherwise resembling a Boston brace, whose defining characteristic is that it is bent or curved to one side—the side being in the opposite direction of the patient's scoliosis curve. Thus, while the patient is wearing the Charleston brace, his or her torso is physically pushed to curve in the opposite direction of his or her natural scoliosis curve, thereby "correcting" the scoliosis curvature during the time when the patient is wearing the brace. Naturally, a patient is incapable of wearing a Charleston brace during the day because the brace forces the patient into a "bent-over" position that would be both awkward in the context of daily life and prohibitive during daily activities. Patients who wear a Charleston brace should be observed closely for the development or increase of compensatory curves. For instance, if a patient's primary curve is a right thoracic curve, the Charleston brace will be constructed to force the patient's spine to bend to the left. While this treatment fares well with the right thoracic curve, it threatens the formation of a left lumbar curve (or an increase in one that is already existent). Accordingly, the Charleston brace should only be considered appropriate treatment for single lumbar or single thoracolumbar curves, whose degree measurements are relatively small. In all other cases, studies have shown that the wearing of a Boston brace is more effective than the wearing of a Charleston brace, for the Boston brace caters to the entire back and is not designed to just counteract a single curve.

THE CRAFTING OF THE BRACE

Though the molded plastic parts of all back braces tend to resemble a generic human figure, not all braces are exactly alike. The majority of back braces are modeled for the patient's body and are designed especially to correct the patient's unique curve. When your doctor tells you that you need to be braced, you will most likely be given the name of an orthotist—a specially trained professional who will actually make the brace. Then, on a separate occasion, you will visit the orthotist to be fitted for your brace. In fitting you for a brace, the orthotist first wraps a gauze material around your torso while you are standing upright. The orthotist then wets this special gauze, and the gauze hardens as it dries, forming a plaster body cast in the exact shape of your body. Once you have been freed from the body cast (in a matter of minutes) and have left the orthotist's office, the orthotist fills the hollow cast with a material that will take the shape of your body. Finally, the orthotist molds the plastic to fit the figure he has crafted to resemble your body; it is in this fashion that the orthotist creates a brace which is handcrafted for and unique to the patient's own body.

When you return to the orthotist's office to obtain your new back brace, it is a good idea to try your brace on. That way, if you find that you are uncomfortable, your orthotist can immediately make any changes or adjustments that will provide you with more comfort.

I still remember the day when I received my back brace. When I tried the brace on for the first time, I remember feeling hot, uncomfortable, and short of breath. The hard, plastic brace was unpleasantly taut on my body. I assumed, though, that I would get used to the brace as I wore it. What I would not get used to, however, was the pain I felt under my arms. My brace came up quite high under my arms so that its edges jabbed into my skin and scraped me whenever I moved. I mentioned this to my orthotist, and he promptly removed the brace and took it into his work room. When he returned, I put the brace on once again; the parts under my arms had been cut so that they were lower and filed so that they were smoother, and I felt absolutely no pain under my arms.

So, if ever you feel notably uncomfortable in your brace, you should not tacitly endure the pain. Instead, tell either your orthotist or your doctor about the problem. Remember, the purpose of a scoliosis back brace is not to hurt you; it is, rather, to help you. You may wonder what is appropriate and what is not appropriate when it comes to complaining about your back brace, for the term "comfort" is purely subjective. But only you can determine when you are comfortable and when you are uncomfortable. Granted, wearing a back brace is not going to be a pleasurable experience and you are going to encounter some rubbing of your skin against the brace, slight shortness of breath, and some sweatiness; however, you should not ignore annoyances such as a jagged brace edge or a single source of constant, unbearable pain. Try not to be a wimp or a complainer about your brace, but do not attempt to be unreasonably tough or invincible either.

Not only do braces come in different styles and shapes, but they come in different colors. Normally, braces come in subtle off-white that hides nicely under any color clothing. However, some people prefer colored braces. If interested, ask your orthotist about the possibility of having a colored brace. I've seen dark blue, baby blue, hot pink, and red braces over the years. Sometimes color can be a useful tool in attracting a child to his or her back brace; after all, a bright, colorful apparatus may seem more fun and enticing to a young scoliosis patient than a sterile-looking, off-white orthosis.

LIVING IN A BRACE: IS IT WORTHWHILE?

Attitudes toward bracing differ greatly among scoliosis patients and doctors alike, and studies testing the effectiveness of various bracing plans continue to be conducted. For effective brace wear, full-time bracing (*i.e.*, twenty-two to twenty-three hours a day) has been shown in long-term studies to be very effective, yielding up to 75 to 80 percent success. Advocates of part-time bracing (*i.e.*, twelve to sixteen hours a day) claim equal results to full-time bracing. However, this has not been proven by any large or reputable studies. As a general rule, you should wear your brace (not including the Charleston brace) for as many hours per day as possible. Most doctors will say that the more hours you wear your brace, the better chance you have of delaying or halting the progression of your scoliosis curve. When it comes to bracing, effectiveness is most often a direct result of time worn.

In my opinion, making occasional excuses for failing to wear your brace for the prescribed amount of time is acceptable. But be careful and use discretion in making your decisions, because making frequent excuses can be detrimental. Just like any other discipline, such as exercising or dieting, bracing can be effective with a "mostly" compliant approach about it. If, however, you make too many excuses and stray too far from the prescribed treatment regimen, your brace will not be effective, and you will inevitably regret it later on. Comparing bracing to some other discipline may enable you to view your adherence to the prescribed treatment in a more objective light. For instance, if you were dieting, you might eat a piece of cake at an occasion like your daughter's wedding. You would not, however, allow yourself to eat cake for no apparent reason or as frequently as every week or two. Similarly, you may remove your brace on given occasions when you really do not want to be inhibited by having to wear it; just try not to get out of hand with discarding your brace.

In general, braces can be removed for activities such as bathing and swimming; even doctors will admit that. But doctors may advise you to keep your brace on during sports, school dances, and other activities. Despite this, many kids and teenagers will remove their braces for such occasions—even if it means lying to their parents about whether they were wearing their braces. As a general rule, you should listen to your doctor, for he or she knows the most about scoliosis and bracing. And, in fact, many young people wear the scoliosis brace with no problem at all. But the truth of the matter is that your doctor is not the one wearing the brace. Living in a back brace is a task that is more easily spoken about than accomplished. It requires you to have an ability to hope for the best and to trust that the brace will work. You are never completely sure whether a brace will be effective; furthermore, in some cases, the brace *is* effective, yet you will still require surgery. This being the case, you should applaud yourself for having the faith and perseverance to wear a back brace in the first place. And while you should continue intensive wear of your back brace, do not feel bad about making some exceptions for yourself or giving yourself some (very limited) "time off" from bracing as a personal reward. Be honest and rational in your approach to brace wear. After all, you are not wearing the brace to please or to aid anyone else; you are wearing it to help yourself and to maintain your own health. In all respects, if you are too active and are out of the brace more than the prescribed hours, then consult your physician for advice. Some activities may have to be curtailed.

A PATIENT'S REACTION TO BRACING

When it comes to treating scoliosis, many patients would rather attempt to halt the progression of their scoliosis curves with back braces than opt immediately for surgery. Because brace wear may seem considerably easier, both physically and financially, than surgery, patients often tend to try it before they resort to spinal fusions. Not all patients, however, view bracing as the easier mode of treatment. Wearing a brace—be it at night only, or for twenty-three hours each day—can take a toll on the comfort, lifestyle, and self-image of a scoliosis patient. Therefore, while many patients faithfully wear back braces, some patients decide either to have surgery immediately or to allow their scoliosis curves to progress to a degree that calls for surgery. While some people are willing to try anything that may improve their condition and postpone or prevent surgery, others assume that surgery is inevitable and that brace wearing is, therefore, an exercise in futility.

Both the patients who choose to wear braces and those who do so grudgingly may find it difficult to adhere to the prescribed treatment once they begin it. Consequently, compliance with bracing may become a problem for the young patient. It may also become a continuing concern for parents who want to say and do the right thing in their encouragement. In order to increase the chances that their children and teenagers will adhere to their prescribed bracing regimens, parents must take a close look at their child's situation and try their best to understand what their child is going through.

From the young patient's point of view, bracing can result in feelings and emotions ranging from mild to intense. For some, the response may be acceptance of the treatment program and resignation to the daily brace-wearing schedule. Other patients may feel hopelessly embarrassed, awkward, and unattractive with their braces on. These types of feelings are especially difficult for adolescents who, as a general rule, never want to present themselves as being different from their peers. Questions such as, "How can I look attractive when I'm wearing this thing?" or "Will anyone ask me out on a date?" or "Can I continue with all my activities now that I am wearing a brace?" or "What did I do to deserve this?" may arise. Worse still, the questions may never be spoken. They may become private and even shame-filled concerns that tear at the fabric of a positive, healthy self-esteem.

The most important element in easing a young scoliosis patient into wearing a back brace may very well be speaking about the scoliosis and the brace. Though it may be difficult at first, discussion of these issues will eventually become more relaxed and helpful. Whatever the case, do not avoid the subjects of scoliosis and the back brace; bring them up frequently to acclimate them into everyday discussion. If a child's or teenager's scoliosis is a secret, he or she will only feel shame, embarrassment, and guilt; if scoliosis and brace wearing are subjects that people are willing to address in casual conversation, the patient is much more likely to feel comfortable with his or her scoliosis and back brace.

STOPS ALONG THE WAY

During the time that you are in your brace, your orthotist will probably ask you to come in for an office visit every four to six months. Each time you visit, your spine will have become used to a new level of being pushed straight, so each time you visit, your orthotist will tighten the pads inside your brace, forcing your spine into an even straighter position. Every brace-tightening feels uncomfortable at first because you are not used to your brace being so tight. But by the time you return to your orthotist for your next tightening, you will be completely used to the old level of tightness and ready to graduate to a new one.

Your doctor will most likely request an office visit every three to four months while you are in your brace (unless there is an isolated problem between visits that causes you to contact your doctor). These doctor's visits are simple checkups to make sure that the brace is working and to address any questions or concerns. X rays may be required during these visits to document the effectiveness of the brace.

HOW LONG DOES BRACING LAST?

Brace wear is continued until you have reached skeletal maturity, as determined by indicators including the Risser sign, menarchal status, and stabilization of height. Some people wear their braces for only a year; others wear their braces for six years. The amount of time you are in the brace depends on your age, curve magnitude, and skeletal maturity upon diagnosis, at the beginning of your time in a brace. Once you stop growing, your doctor will tell you to wean yourself from the brace over a six to twelve month period. This weaning process, which entails wearing the brace for, perhaps, a few hours less each week, is very important. An abrupt discarding of the brace may result in back pain (for the patient is not accustomed to being unsupported), or an increase in the curve that may have been prevented.

I am a definite advocate of the weaning process, as my own doctor failed to warn me about weaning. As I neared the end of my brace wear, I was to go to France to participate in an international summer dance program. I asked my doctor if he thought I should take my brace with me.

"No," he said. "You're almost done growing, and I don't think it will make a difference." Naturally believing what my doctor said, I moved from wearing the brace all day, every day to being in France for three straight weeks and not wearing my brace at all. At first I felt happy; my body was free! After about three days, though, I began to experience severe muscle pain. The pain got to be so unbearable that I sought the treatment of a French physiotherapist. He maneuvered my spine and gave me muscle stimulation to relieve the pain.

As it turned out, my scoliosis increased about five degrees over the course of that summer. When I returned to America and sought advice from a different doctor, I found out that I had not, in fact, completed my growth at the *beginning* of the summer. *During* the summer months, I had just been completing my adolescent growth spurt, and I should have been wearing a brace the entire time. The pain I had experienced, the new doctor told me, was a joint result of the fact that I had not been ready to stop wearing the brace and the fact that I did not wean myself from the brace; it was then that I learned what weaning is in regard to bracing.

Given the chance to go back in time and repeat my steps, I would definitely have taken my brace to France, and I would have slowly weaned myself from it once I had *completely* finished growing. I regret that my doctor misjudged my skeletal maturity and that he failed to tell me about weaning, and I regret that I had to pay the consequence (progression of my scoliosis) for his miscalculations.

A General Outlook on Bracing

Although, when it comes to bracing, doctors' opinions vary and patients' attitudes vacillate, anyone would be remiss to forget that bracing has been shown in innumerable studies sponsored by very reputable sources to be effective. If worn continuously and for the prescribed number of hours, braces work well in growing patients whose curves range from twenty to forty degrees. While they do not correct scoliosis, braces certainly slow and sometimes stop scoliosis curves from progressing to higher degrees of curvature. So the decision of whether to wear a brace and hope to prevent (or at least to delay) the need for surgery, or to wait patiently for your scoliosis curve to reach a degree that requires surgery is ultimately yours. If you are a candidate for bracing, try not to lose sight of the fact that bracing is a privilege not available to all scoliosis patients. Some people have curves that cannot be controlled by bracing; some have only moderate curves but are too old to try bracing; and some just need surgery right away. But you have the chance to wear a brace and to try to prevent surgery. Do not take it for granted.

SELF-ESTEEM AND BODY IMAGE

Self-esteem is the result of a realistic and healthy level of self-regard and a sense of self-appreciation. It is a way of thinking, feeling, and acting that implies we accept, trust, respect, and believe in ourselves. It is a personal judgement of worthiness expressed in attitudes that a person holds toward himself or herself.

Psychologists profess that self-esteem is essential for any human being's psychological survival. People who constantly judge and reject themselves can have a diminished sense of their personal power and self-effectiveness. Low self-esteem has been found in almost all problematic psychological conditions that can appear in childhood and adolescence. In later years, adults with low self-esteem may take on fewer social, educational, and career risks for fear of rejection. They may have difficulty meeting people, interviewing for jobs, and testing their own limits. They may avoid being the center of attention or have difficulty hearing criticism, asking for help, expressing sexuality, and solving life's problems. As such, self-esteem is important throughout one's entire life.

For adolescents, self-esteem is intimately interwoven with physical appearance, body image, and acceptance among peers. During the teen years, body shape, coordination, sexual characteristics, appetite, weight, and height all change drastically, and adolescents tend to be very sensitive to these physical changes. Many are constantly comparing themselves to their peers and to images readily available in media and advertising. In such comparisons, adolescents wearing braces may come up short if they focus only on physicality. Thoughts about having scoliosis and wearing a brace—such as "What will my friends say?" or "Scoliosis only happens to rejects," or "How can any guy/girl be attracted to me?"—can become the core of an isolated, alienated, unlovable, and unworthy "I'm not okay" self-image. This problem is compounded for those individuals who are already critical and perfectionistic regarding appearance, achievement, and abilities. Furthermore, adolescents with scoliosis—especially those who have to wear back braces—are likely to feel different, and therefore isolated, from their peers. At a time in one's life when one's affiliation with some sort of group (be it a sports team, a band, or an arbitrary group of friends) is crucial and one's identity has yet to solidify, having scoliosis or having to wear a brace can set someone apart from the crowd in a way that is unfavorable. Adolescents with scoliosis often feel very isolated and alone—as if there were no one for them to identify with or relate to. These feelings can contribute to melancholy and a low self-esteem.

A study published in 1994 showed that young adults who had been adolescent idiopathic scoliosis patients had a notably higher prevalence of self-reported arthritis than control subjects who did not have scoliosis. Scoliosis subjects perceived themselves to be less healthy than their peers and had a poorer perception of body image.

Without the added pressure of dealing with scoliosis, adolescence can be a difficult time in a person's life. Teenagers must endure unfamiliar changes in their bodies, awkward phases, and scrutiny from peers on an everyday basis. Adding the element of scoliosis—and perhaps a back brace or an embarrassing rib hump—to a teenage life can upset the fragile emotional balance that the teenager strives, throughout adolescence, to maintain. Figuring out how to deal with the problems that a back brace may cause an adolescent and finding a way to boost an adolescent scoliosis patient's self-esteem are, therefore, very important tasks to accomplish.

I still vividly remember the height of my own adolescent angst. When I first got my back brace, during the August preceding my freshman year in high school, I was terribly distressed. I didn't know what to do. I wanted to make a good impression on the new kids I would meet, to wear clothes that were stylish and sometimes form-fitting, and to appear like a "normal" teenager. But now I had to decide how I was going to handle having this burdensome back brace. Ultimately, I decided to be very open and honest about my scoliosis with friends and teachers at school. I came to the conclusion that ignorance breeds cruelty and false gossip in a high school setting. I realized that if the kids at school saw some strange *thing* lurking under my deliberately baggy clothing, they would draw their own conclusions and create rumors about what this "thing" was for, in order to satisfy their own fears and curiosities. I combated this possibility by telling everyone, outright, that I had scoliosis, a curvature of the spine, that I had to wear this back brace, and that I felt perfectly normal and fine. This way, no one could talk about me behind my back; I made everyone comfortable enough to speculate and ask questions right in front of me. Luckily, my peers and elders reacted well to the way in which I handled my scoliosis and my brace. They were, for the most part, kind, understanding, and sympathetic.

My psychological comfort level was greatly enhanced by the reactions and support of a few instrumental people. My advisor (the equivalent of a homeroom teacher) at school, for one, was very accepting of my scoliosis. I remember that when he went around my advisor group

TEN WAYS TO BOOST YOUR SELF ESTEEM

1. See yourself accurately. We all have strengths and assets, together with shortcomings. Focus on the strengths and assets.
2. Recognize the ways you put yourself down and criticize yourself. Replace these negative self-statements with self-praising affirmations. Actually say the affirmations.
3. Reward yourself when you've done a good job, coped with a difficult situation, or handled stress well.
4. Learn how to ask for what you need and how to say "no" to those things you don't. This may take some practice.
5. Accept your body—all of it! When you look into a mirror, don't just focus on your back or your hip. See all of yourself, not parts in isolation from your whole self.
6. Don't let scoliosis define you. You are more, much more than your scoliosis or any physical condition.
7. Set goals for yourself—goals that are realistic and healthy. Make daily progress toward those goals. Praise yourself for your progress.
8. Respect yourself. Be your own best friend.
9. Discover your "shoulds." Are they realistic? Where did you learn them? Replace them if they are unrealistic, perfectionistic, or unhealthy.
10. Learn to laugh and learn to smile. Life isn't all serious. Discover again how to enjoy it.

of seven kids on the first day of school, asking what each of us had done that summer, I told everyone that I had gotten a back brace. As I took the first step of sharing my scoliosis experience with my peers, my advisor supported me by asking questions and encouraging interest and acceptance among the rest of the group. He expressed admiration for the courage and vivacity I had maintained despite my difficult situation, and I appreciated that more than I realized at the time. Reactions like this, whether they are expressed through looks or spoken words, can make all the difference to someone wearing a brace. Friends and teachers of a person in a brace can be supportive just by expressing interest in and concern for that person and his or her condition.

Each child or adolescent who has scoliosis or who has to wear a back brace must decide how to deal with the scoliosis and the back brace in a way that will best suit him or her. Remember, it is generally true that you can influence people's reactions by exuding your own distinct attitude. If you maintain a high level of self-esteem and inner strength, people will sense it in your presence and will be less likely to deprecate or poke fun at your scoliosis or your brace.

Personally, after an awkward adjustment period, I became very comfortable with my brace and my self-image. I thought nothing was wrong with my appearance, and I tried to live life as if I weren't even wearing a brace. The overwhelming sense of normalcy that permeated my life in my brace, however, was interrupted on certain occasions. For instance, when I wore overalls over my brace, the task of going to the bathroom was a difficult one. Not only did I have to undo the overalls, but I had to figure out a way to move the brace underneath. As I would struggle with my garments—cloth and plastic alike—in a stall in the girls' bathroom, my friends would tarry by the sinks, waiting for me.

"Brooke, are you okay in there?" they would ask me, laughing, after about ten minutes.

"Sure," I would say. "I'll be right out. It's just that I'm wearing overalls *and* my brace today, so I'm having a bit of difficulty in here . . . hold on." Of course I got used to maneuvering things after some practice, and my friends got used to waiting for me. But the bathroom was one of the few places where I really noticed that my scoliosis and my back brace made me different from my friends. Feeling different didn't matter too much to me, because my friends accepted my difference and addressed it as a nonissue. This, too, can be a way for friends, teachers, and family members of a brace-wearer to ease the feelings of the person in the brace. By accepting a friend's or student's brace, getting over it, and acting as if it is not there, people can make a brace-wearer feel like less of a standout amongst peers. This, in turn, can improve the brace-wearer's self esteem.

One particular occasion comes to mind every time I think about my own self-image. One night I was sitting in my bedroom diligently doing my homework. I decided that I needed a study break, so I walked downstairs into the kitchen, where I met my parents and my brother. Greeting them casually, I continued to the refrigerator for a snack. But before I opened the refrigerator door, my parents and brother burst out in laughter.

"What?" I asked, turning to face them.

"God, Brooke!" my father said. "Look at yourself!"

"If only your friends could see you now!" my brother added.

At first, I had no idea what they were alluding to. When I walked over to the oven to look at my reflection in the shiny black door, however, I, too, began to laugh. There I was, the epitome of the aesthetically challenged adolescent girl; I was wearing my big, goofy, fuzzy slippers, a pair of baggy plaid pajama pants that were pulled up high on my waist (over the lower part of my back brace), and a faded, bleach-stained baby blue tank top beneath the uncovered mass of plastic that enveloped my body. My disheveled ponytail, my glasses, my retainers, and the white spots on my face (from where I had applied acne medication) completed the comical picture. In retrospect, I could have been very upset by the way I looked that night—and at that stage of my life—but I found it easier and more uplifting just to laugh about it.

Sometimes when people must face upsetting truths, such as having scoliosis and having to wear a back brace at a very difficult time in one's life, the only effective remedy is humor. I've found that laughing at yourself and at your problems makes them seem less severe, and it lets people know that *you* are not the problem. The acts of laughing at, recognizing, and talking about the problem show others that you regard the problem as its own entity; though it may affect you, it has not become you.

If, while in the midst of a problem, you tell yourself that the problem will eventually fade, you will feel a lot better about yourself and your life. If you treat your condition wisely, be it by wearing a brace or having surgery, you should know that your decision is not hurting you, it is improving your health. And if you exude confidence in the midst of adversity, others will have no chance to mock or feel pity for you; they will admire you for your courage. As soon as you develop a strong sense of self-confidence and learn to emit that confidence to others, your shining personality will eclipse the back brace you are wearing.

COMPLIANCE ISSUES AND CONSEQUENCES

Before investing approximately $2,000 and all of your hopes in a back brace, you should address the issue of compliance honestly and realistically. Parents and children will benefit from having an honest discussion, perhaps with their doctor, about whether the person with scoliosis will really be able to adhere to the prescribed amount of brace wear.

Many teenagers accept the diagnosis of scoliosis and bracing and, without much difficulty, follow through with the daily bracing schedule as prescribed. Others may have more difficulty, including partial, intermittent, or no compliance whatsoever. Some refuse to wear the brace right from the start. Younger children who are used to doing as they are told may wear the brace, but may have very strong feelings of resentment toward it. Clues indicating that a child or teenager suffers from these sorts of feelings include expressed apprehensions, excessive worry or anxiety, self-critical statements, concerns about the future, and avoidance of social situations and friends. Falling school grades, various physical complaints, increasing school absences, changes in eating or sleeping habits, irritability and moodiness, and the onset of fears and phobias are also possible signs that your son or daughter is having trouble complying with his or her bracing regimen. If children or teenagers notice that they are having serious trouble with brace wear, they should honestly express their feelings to a parent or doctor; if parents notice that their children are having trouble with brace wearing, they should try to broach the subject with them and attempt to get to the root of the problem.

Both parents and children should know that degree of compliance to the prescribed brace treatment plays a major role in determining the effectiveness of a brace. While this fact suggests that adherence to brace treatment is an utterly simple issue, the issue is simultaneously simple and complex. It is simple in that the patient has a clear-cut decision to make between agreeing to wear the back brace and deciding not to wear it; it is complex in that if a patient does choose to wear a back brace, there is no guarantee that the brace will be effective.

While braces are effective in most cases, they are not effective in all cases. Therefore, any number of things can happen to a patient involved with bracing. The patient may wear the brace for several years and, if his or her curve stops progressing once skeletal maturity has been reached, surgery may be avoided. The patient who faithfully wears the brace may also end up needing surgery if the curve continues to progress after skeletal maturity has been reached.

My friend Kerrith, a talkative redhead with a quick wit and a passion for dance, began wearing her brace when she was in the seventh grade. Though she has gone through difficult phases of hating her brace, trying to burn and destroy it, and lying to her parents about wearing it, she has, over the years, grown to be a faithful brace wearer. Consequently, Kerrith's curve has been controlled quite nicely. The rapid curve progression that had begun at the beginning of her adolescent growth period was halted by her wearing the brace. Now that she is seventeen and has reached skeletal maturity, Kerrith's curve has stopped progressing. Frozen at a harmlessly low degree of curvature, her spine will never require surgery. If she had not worn her brace for so many years, her curve just might have progressed to a degree that would have required surgery.

I, too, was a faithful brace wearer, but I ended up in a position quite different than Kerrith's. I wore my brace faithfully for a period of one year (from the time when it was diagnosed to the time when I stopped growing), hoping, all the while, to prevent my two scoliosis curves from progressing. For that short period of time, the degree measures of my curves remained constant. After I reached skeletal maturity, though, my curves continued to progress. The doctors expect my spine to continue to curve at a rate of about one degree per year, for the rest of my life, until surgery. In retrospect, I do not regret having worn the brace, because if I had not worn it, my curves might have been much more severe today. Nevertheless, I regret that the progression of my scoliosis curves did not stop when my bones stopped growing.

On the other hand, patients who opt not to disrupt their lives by wearing the brace may stop progressing at skeletal maturity and never need surgery (though this scenario is highly unlikely). Most members of this noncompliant group do end up needing surgery, yet the majority here is not upset by their having to have surgery; they made a conscious decision to evade brace wearing, and they were prepared to deal with whatever consequences their rapidly progressing scoliosis curves would elicit.

Most, if not all, doctors advocate brace wear when it is a viable option, but once patients have left the doctor's office, adherence to the prescribed wear is up to them. If a patient is honestly adherent to bracing and wears his or her brace for the recommended number of hours each day, the brace is likely to be effective; if a patient is either openly or secretly noncompliant to brace treatment, the brace will not work. The majority of "braceable" scoliosis patients agree to try brace-wearing.

Some patients *really* prefer not to wear back braces and decide to have

REASONS WHY SOMEONE MIGHT NOT ADHERE TO A SUGGESTED TREATMENT REGIMEN

1. I spend too much time participating in a sport or activity, and I would not want a back brace to interfere with my devotion to that sport or activity.
2. I really don't care about the progression of my scoliosis and, instead of wearing a brace, I would prefer to have surgery.
3. I absolutely refuse to wear a brace to school or in a social setting.
4. I am worried about my appearance in a brace.
5. I worry that my friend(s) or boyfriend/girlfriend won't like me if I wear a brace.
6. I receive no support at home, and I cannot handle brace-wearing by myself.
7. Considering my lifestyle, brace-wearing is just not realistic.
8. I am embarrassed about my scoliosis, and I feel stupid/silly/humiliated wearing a brace.

QUESTIONS TO ASK YOURSELF WHEN CONTEMPLATING BRACING

1. Will I really be committed to wearing this brace, even when it is difficult or when I get fed up with it?
2. Is eighteen to twenty-three hours of brace-wear per day realistic, considering my lifestyle and daily schedule?
3. Am I willing to make sacrifices so that I can wear my brace and treat my scoliosis?
4. Will I get discouraged when I run into minor problems or difficulties with my brace?
5. Will my family be supportive and understanding of bracing?
6. Can I find the strength to stand up to people who aren't understanding?
7. Is the parent-child-doctor relationship honest enough so that I will feel comfortable being honest about any problems I am having with the brace?
8. Will my parents be capable of disciplining me and rationally guiding me through the duration of my time in a brace?

surgery immediately. Most of the time, these are people who are borderline surgical candidates anyway, who find that they cannot comply with brace wear for reasons ranging from being overweight to being critically embarrassed by a brace in a social setting. Before you jump into surgery, though, you should realize that surgery is a huge undertaking that encompasses time spent in the hospital, considerable pain, and a long recovery period. In weighing possibilities for treatment of scoliosis, you and your parents should examine both bracing and surgery thoroughly; visit several doctors to obtain a wide range of opinions and, ultimately, choose whichever treatment will be most beneficial to you.

FAMILIAL ANXIETY AND ACCEPTANCE

The family is a big factor in determining whether to brace a child and whether the child will receive the support he or she needs to continue wearing the brace. Orthopedic surgeons, mental health professionals, and patients agree that the way a person's family acts toward that person's scoliosis brace directly affects the person's own feelings about his or her brace.

Parents may have a range of reactions to their child's initial diagnosis and subsequent need to wear a brace. In their concern about potential health issues and cosmetic deformities in their child, parents may experience disappointment, sadness, anxiety, anger, confusion, or even depression. In error, they might blame themselves for their child's condition. Some marriages may be quite strained by the prolonged stress of the child's condition. The parents may experience the diagnosis of scoliosis and subsequent bracing as traumatic events for themselves and their child. Mothers as primary caretakers may be especially affected in trying to monitor the daily bracing regimen; fathers may feel inadequate and less than competent to cope. Some couples may just not know how to talk to each other about how they feel. And prior marital disharmony may exacerbate the problem. These family patterns can result in detrimental approaches to the child's psychological health. The most common of these patterns include overanxious and overprotective approaches, overindulgent approaches, overcontrolling and rigid approaches, resentment and rejection of the child, disinterest, and neglect. These types of scenarios present the worst environments for children and teenagers who are wearing braces. Not only do these child-

---

THREE THINGS PARENTS CAN DO
TO MAKE BRACING EASIER

1. Buy your child some new clothes when he or she gets a brace. Getting clothes to fit over, and perhaps to hide, the brace may make brace-wearing altogether more exciting and tolerable.

2. Act according to the way your child acts. Children and teenagers with back braces may shift moods from day to day. One day, they may need your sympathy; another day, they may need you to ignore the brace and act as if they aren't wearing it.

3. Be supportive. Give your child periodic words of encouragement to let him or her know that his or her brace-wearing is not going unnoticed and unappreciated.

---

ren and teenagers have to handle wearing back braces, but they have to handle their difficult home situations as well—and this can make brace-wearing virtually impossible to all those except the strongest, most determined, young patients. Doctors are reluctant to recommend bracing if there is a perception involving a difficult home situation and lack of family support, as these patients frequently become noncompliant.

Luckily, most parents will rely on already well-developed communication skills to share their feelings with one another. Together, they will create a consistent, empathetic, and supportive approach to their child's efforts. In addition, they will talk to siblings of the affected child and explain to them the issues of scoliosis and bracing. Hopefully the siblings, too, will grow to understand and behave in ways that accomodate the affected child's condition. Creating this type of comfortable home environment while maintaining a fairly normal home life and family balance (*i.e.*, avoiding treating the affected child as if he or she cannot function independently, focusing on him or her too much and neglecting other children in the family, or acting overly sympathetic) will provide the best and most salutary medium for a child or teenager affected with scoliosis and wearing a brace. Familial support and encouragement may just push an otherwise resentful child or teenager toward willing compliance.

CREATIVE COPING TECHNIQUES AND EXERCISES

Once an individual has gotten his or her brace, he or she inevitably wonders how to go about living with it. A person may be psychologically and emotionally comfortable with the idea of having to wear a brace, yet the physical aspect of brace-wearing may remain a problem to be reckoned with. I remember the first few weeks of my brace-wearing days; I could not sleep, wear my normal clothes, pick things up off the floor, or breathe freely. Yet, as time passed, I slowly became aware of things I could do to make my new "life in a brace" less arduous. Despite the initial difficulties that accompany brace-wearing, most people quickly become used to their braces, adding unique tricks and tips to their repertoires as they become seasoned with experience and metamorphose into brace-wearing virtuosos.

Some younger children may want to decorate their braces with stickers and colored markers; others may wish to name their braces, thereby allowing the braces to adopt their own personalities. It is through these creative mediums that uncomfortable, repellent back braces can become fun, attractive pieces of art or healthful, helpful companions.

In addressing a teen's coping with brace-wearing, it is crucial to address and demystify the common act of "back-cracking." A few years ago, I began cracking my back (an act similar to cracking one's knuckles). Twisting from side to side, I would listen for a series of popping sounds accompanied by an immediate looser feeling in my vertabrae. Then, when I began wearing a back brace for my scoliosis, I became quite skilled at the art of back-cracking. One morning, I awoke and sat straight up. Removing my brace, as I did every morning when I woke up, I felt a distinct stiffness in my back; the stiffness was undoubtedly a result of my having slept for eight hours in a brace that held my spine still in a single position. Instinctively, I began twisting from side to side, waiting for my vertabrae to make popping sounds and hoping to restore some sort of flexibility to my rigid spine. All of a sudden, I felt my vertabrae start to loosen, one by one, and I heard a symphony of popping and cracking sounds; I had never heard anything like it before. Since then, I've become a habitual back-cracker. And, in my experience with other scoliosis patients, I've come to realize that I am not alone in my tendency to crack my back. Though many people with (and without) scoliosis crack their backs on a daily basis, they all seem to be concerned as to whether this back-cracking is harmful to their spines or to their general health. In my own curiosity, I have asked various doctors for their opinions on the matter. The doctors I have asked have answered that the act of cracking one's back is analogous to the act of cracking one's knuckles; it releases excess nitrogen that gets stuck between one's joints. Back-cracking is in no way harmful to one's health, unless it causes noticeable pain. Furthermore, contrary to certain rumors and myths that have been generated over time, your spine will not break, crack, or get bigger if you crack it. People who crack their backs need not worry about doing so unless they are forcing themselves to do so unnecessarily or they are feeling pain when they do so.

Beyond cracking your back, there are many things that you can do to enhance your comfort while you are wearing a back brace. If the brace makes you hot and sweaty, use talcum powder and wear cotton undershirts. Talcum powder will soften your skin and help to prevent excessive perspiring while you are in the brace. You should *always* wear something underneath your brace to prevent chafing and irritation. Thin, fitted cotton undershirts (either tank, short-sleeved, or long-sleeved—whichever you prefer) tend to work well under braces for several reasons: they maintain skin coolness by allowing air to pass through them; they do not bunch up and form bulges of fabric that press into your skin when placed underneath a brace; and they absorb perspiration quite well. In addition, all outer garments, such as pants and skirts, should be worn on top of the brace. Females may or may not want to wear bras under their braces. Sometimes braces are binding and supportive enough to replace bras; however, for an individual who wishes to wear one, a bra should be worn beneath the cotton undershirt. Females usually prefer simpler bras (*i.e.*, sports bras) that lack any decoration, metal hooks, and strap adjusters (these elements of some bras tend to dig into the skin when placed beneath a tight-fitting back brace). Finally, females wearing Milwaukee braces should take care to wear their hair in a ponytail, bun, or some other "updo." Hair getting caught in the neck ring of Milwaukee braces can prove to be both annoying and painful.

In terms of activities, sleeping and bending down can be among the most difficult for a brace wearer. When wearing a brace, it is often difficult to sleep on your stomach because you are unable to turn your head to one side. The first night I slept with my brace on, I instinctively tried to lay facedown, with my head turned sideways; I realized that my normal sleeping position was impossible to achieve while wearing my brace when I found myself unable to turn my head far enough to either side. Much to my dismay, my brace only allowed me to plant my face directly into my pillow. Rather than smothering myself, I learned to sleep on my back and on my sides. Getting used to sleeping with my brace on took a full seven to ten days; it was not easy. But my stubborn persistence and unwillingness to remove my brace paid off; eventually I was as comfortable sleeping with my brace on as I was sleeping with it off. I had a similar learning experience when I first tried to pick something up off the floor while wearing my brace. In math class one day, I dropped my pencil. Naturally, I leaned over to retrieve it, but when my hand was about six inches from the floor, it stopped! I could not physically reach any further without tipping my body so much as to knock myself out of my chair. Not wanting to slide out of my chair and onto the floor in a desperate attempt to grab my pencil, I asked a friend sitting nearby to retrieve my pencil for me. After that episode, I schemed until I found a way to pick things up off the ground; after all, I was not about to become dependent on other people's help for the duration of my time in my back brace. I realized that, since I absolutely could not bend over, I would have to squat. From then on, I never again had trouble reaching the floor. When my pencil dropped in math class, I would quickly stand up, bend my legs (while keeping my braced torso straight) until my dangling fingers brushed the floor so I could discreetly grab my pencil and slide back into my desk chair.

While the aforementioned coping techniques are geared toward physical comfort, there also exist many coping techniques that involve physical appearance. Large, baggy apparel is the best clothing option for concealing back braces. Pants and skirts with either elastic waists or one or two sizes larger than your regular size allow you some extra room for the fraction of an inch that the brace adds to your waistline. Baggy or billowing shirts will also help conceal the presence of a back brace. Regardless of the clothes you decide to wear atop your brace, you should remember that most people will never even know you are wearing a brace (it is much more apparent to you than it is to others); on the other hand, some aspects of braces, such as the neck rings of Milwaukee braces and the high-reaching tops of the back portions of Boston TLSO braces, are aspects that are likely to be noticed, no matter what you are wearing. So, if concealing your brace is important to you, you can easily be about 90 percent successful in doing so.

BROOKE

By the time I had obtained my brace, it was late August of 1995. That September, I began my freshman year in high school. I forced myself to wear the brace for the required eighteen hours each day, regardless of how hot or uncomfortable it made me feel. In fact, I sometimes made myself wear the brace for up to twenty or twenty-one hours on a given day, just to give myself the advantage of having extra treatment. The only times when I took my brace off were at daily ballet classes and certain special occasions.

Soon after I had gotten my brace, I found baggy clothing that hid it quite well. Most of the time, people didn't even know that I was wearing the brace. I also developed tricks to make myself more comfortable and to enable myself to walk and function without looking or feeling foolish. And, during the night, I forced myself to become used to sleeping in my brace. Though I had to endure several uncomfortable, sleepless nights at the beginning of my time in the brace, I refused to remove the brace; after all, if I removed it during the night, how would I *ever* be able to sleep in it? My persistence paid off. Within a week, I was able to sleep peacefully in my brace.

If ever I brought up the subject of my scoliosis, I would receive many questions and queries from classmates and teachers alike. No one chided or mocked me for having to wear a brace; they just asked intuitive questions. By being open about my scoliosis and my brace, I eliminated the possibility of having people talk about it behind my back. Most people thought that it was too bad that I had to wear a hot, uncomfortable brace all day, but they also respected and admired the fact that I wasn't afraid to treat my scoliosis.

When the initial interest had abated and classmates had gotten used to my brace, it became somewhat of a joke. While walking down the halls, I would receive numerous punches in the stomach. My friends never hit me very hard, but even if they had, their hands would have hurt more than my stomach, because underneath my baggy clothing lay a hard layer of plastic.

"Ha! I have 'abs of steel'—no, I have *abs of plastic!*" I would joke.

Over time, I learned that my friends, teachers, and family members were not the only ones to whom I had to explain the concepts of scoliosis and bracing. Every Tuesday, I tutored a group of first graders who needed special attention. I had been tutoring the same children at an elementary school for about a year when I got my back brace, so I had already developed close relationships with some of them. One day, two of my favorite kids, Stephanie and Tayanna, grabbed hold of my hands and begged me not to go; I said that I had to go back to my own school and reminded them that I would be back in just one week. I gave Stephanie a hug and suddenly heard her yell, "Ah! What do you have on your back?" She jumped away from me and looked aghast. I then realized that Stephanie had felt my back brace. I laughed, then struggled to find words to explain to this seven-year-old what the brace was for. I pulled my shirt up a bit so the girls could glimpse the plastic brace and see for themselves that I was not some strange sort of bionic girl. Stephanie and Tayanna looked sympathetic after I explained to them that my back was crooked and that the purpose of the brace was to keep it from becoming more crooked. Every Tuesday throughout the rest of the year, the first words I would hear out of Stephanie's and Tayanna's mouths would be, "How's your back, Brooke? Is it better?" I was touched by their conscientious compassion and their interest in my condition. From the moment that I had explained everything to them, these kind first graders were never frightened of or compelled to make fun of my back brace; their understanding, accepting attitudes were, in my opinion, behavioral examples for everyone to follow.

While the things that happened to me when I wore my brace to public places were interesting, my favorite brace-wearing anecdote took place when I was at home. There, I never wore a shirt over my brace; I always wore some sort of undershirt beneath the brace and allowed the brace to be my outermost, visible layer of garb. One day, I walked into the kitchen and found my mother talking over the kitchen counter to our new housekeeper, Mary, who was from Malaysia. I greeted the two women, picked up a can of soda, and returned to my room. Later, my mother came to my room to see me; she was almost unable to speak because she was laughing so hard.

"You'll never guess what Mary said to me after you left the kitchen!" she exclaimed.

"What?"

"After you left, I tried to explain to Mary what your back brace is for—you know, just so that she wouldn't always wonder about it. When I had finished explaining its purpose, she started laughing and told me that she had thought it was some sort of thing American girls wear to make their chests look bigger!"

"Gee, I never thought of it *that* way," I replied. Because my brace was a TLSO, which covered my entire torso from my hips to my underarms and left an open space only in the front, the chest area, Mary had thought that it resembled some sort of bust-enhancing apparatus. I, along with my mother, laughed out loud at the assumption Mary had made.

I stopped wearing my brace one year after I had begun wearing it, when my doctor told me that I was almost fully grown and that I did not have to wear my brace anymore. X rays taken in the months and years after I finished growing showed that, contrary to what I had hoped for, my spine was not frozen at a thirty-six degree thoracic curve and a thirty-nine degree lumbar curve; it was progressing. Three years after my diagnosis, at seventeen, my curves are each approaching fifty degrees, and a few doctors have told me that surgery is necessary. Despite the fact that my curves are increasing with each moment that passes, I remain glad that I wore my brace when I did, because if I had-n't worn it, there is no telling how severe my scoliosis would be today. If I can say anything about my bracing experience, it is that wearing a brace at least bought me some time—perhaps a few years—before I would have to have surgery.

DENISE

In 1972, Denise's doctor informed her, at a routine physical, that she had scoliosis. Noticing an obvious curvature in Denise's spine, the doctor recommended that Denise visit the Newington Children's Hospital in Connecticut to obtain X rays and to determine exactly how serious her scoliosis was. Through a subsequent X-ray session and examination at the hospital, fifteen-year-old Denise learned that she had scoliosis that could be controlled by bracing. Almost immediately, Denise's doctor prescribed a Milwaukee back brace for her.

"It was probably one of the first plastic braces," Denise says. "Before then, they were all leather." The brace consisted of molded plastic and a metal rod that spanned from Denise's lower torso to below her chin.

"I was to wear the brace for twenty-three hours every day," Denise remembers. "I could only take it off for one hour each day, when I wanted to shower." In addition to her back brace, Denise ended up wearing a mouthguard at night. The metal chinpiece component of her brace pushed up the bottom half of her jaw so that her teeth ground together when she was sleeping; the mouthguard prevented this.

Having given her this Milwaukee brace to wear, Denise's doctor told her that she would have few physical restrictions while wearing the brace. Her only limits, he assured her, would be self-inflicted. Therefore, Denise kept herself busy as an active participant in high school activities such as jumping on the trampoline and attending boy-girl mixers, all the while wearing her brace.

Outside school, Denise occupied herself with a job at a shoe store.

"I used to scale the walls in the back room, looking for shoes and everything—with my brace on!" says Denise. "I wanted to hide the brace, though, so I wore cowls, ascots, and sweaters with high necklines even before they were in style—even during the summer. I didn't want to hide my brace because I was *embarrassed* about it; I just didn't want to have to answer to every person who walked into the store."

After several months of working at the same shoe store, Denise got to know the personnel there quite well. She recalls how curious her fellow workers were about her strange clothing choices. Sometimes, they would glimpse metal near Denise's neck or an edge of a plastic bodice under her sweater. Other times, Denise's friends would come into the store and playfully tap her body, creating the sound that a hand banging against hard plastic makes; Denise laughs as she thinks about how this must have baffled her coworkers.

Despite having some physical difficulty, answering some curious questions, and needing to have cysts removed (cysts that had formed because of her brace's constant rubbing against her skin), Denise had few problems with the brace and became an avid brace wearer. She remembers that two particular kids at her high school helped her to realize that she was not the only one in a back brace and that brace-wearing didn't have to be a burden—it might even have been a "cool" thing.

"There was one boy, Sammy, at school who wore a brace and set the precedent for all brace wearers so I didn't have to," says Denise fondly. "And then there was this girl at my friend Billy's house. She was the most beautiful girl I had ever seen, and she wore a brace, too. I admired this girl *and* her brace. In fact, I saw her at a party right before I got my brace and, believe it or not, I kind of wanted a brace after I had seen her."

Denise wore the brace for twenty-three hours every day from the time she was fifteen years old to the time she was seventeen. At seventeen, Denise reached skeletal maturity and was told by her doctor that she should begin to wean herself off of brace wearing.

Since her teenage years, Denise has never had to treat her scoliosis. Her curve stabilized at thirty-five degrees after she had finished grow-

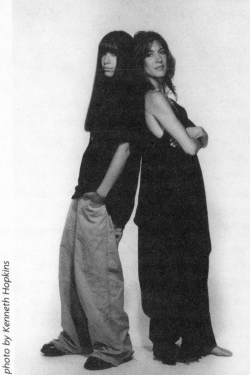

photo by Kenneth Hopkins

Daughter and mother, Erika (left) and Denise (right)—a genetic link.

ing and never required any surgery. Since then, Denise has grown to become a succesful artist and a mother of two. Even at forty, she remains mindful of her back. From exercising each day, to stretching her back, to standing up straight, Denise does everything she can to help her back. She never forgets that she has scoliosis and never rests in her attempts to maintain a strong physique, for she knows that if she lets herself slouch naturally or allows her back muscles to get weak, her degree of spine curvature may increase.

ERIKA

The school bus dropped Erika off at the bottom of the hill. As she walked up that hill, toward her home, she began to feel sharp pains in the muscles in her back; the heavy, book-filled backpack she carried aggravated her condition. But Erika managed to bear the pain until she reached her house. As she walked inside, she broke down and began to cry while repeating the words, "my back hurts, my back hurts." Erika's mother, Denise made her daughter bend over so that she could examine Erika's back. She remembers seeing what looked like "a boomerang shot in two directions."

Five years prior to this episode, Erika had been diagnosed with scoliosis. Denise, who had scoliosis as a teenager, had been eyeing her daughter's spine for years in the hope that she would never detect a curvature. Unfortunately, the spine disorder that had plagued Denise's teenage years had returned to haunt her daughter over twenty years later.

"Well, I looked all the time," she said. "I'd have her [Erika] bend over. At school, they'd look at her back. They were doing that anyway. Everybody said she was fine. I just decided that an X ray would tell me that she was *really* fine. As a mother, I'd feel better. So I took her to Newington [Children's Hospital] where I went for my scoliosis."

When the doctors at the children's hospital saw Erika's X rays, they immediately put her into a back brace. Erika, then just eight years old, had a thirty-five-degree thoracic curve and a twenty-seven-degree lumbar curve. Had her mother not been so vigilant, Erika's curve might have gone undetected for years.

At first, Erika loved her low-profile Boston brace. She proudly wore it all the time. "I used to love it," she remembers. "I used to bully around with the kids. I'd say, 'Come on, punch me!' and they'd be like, 'Ow!' They didn't expect it."

As soon as she had been put into the brace, though, Erika began to grow rapidly. She went through three braces, each a bit larger than its predecessor, within a year. By the time she was nine years old, and wearing her third brace, her attitude had gone from enthusiastic to noncompliant.

"By the third brace," Denise remembers, "Erika said, 'I'm not wearing this thing!' We revisited the doctor and I said, 'I can't get her to wear it. Every day is a battle.'"

Denise couldn't bear to see her daughter in such misery anymore. So, without permission from any doctor, she allowed nine-year-old Erika to stop wearing the brace. For the time being, both Erika and Denise were a lot happier than they had been when Erika was wearing the brace. Life without a back brace—without having to deal with scoliosis—was much easier than life with the brace. Unfortunately, Denise did not consider the potential repercussions of her decision.

"I just thought you wear the brace and it's over. I thought it was something for cosmetics—if you wanted to have a nicer posture, you wear this thing and it'll help you. Erika was going crazy; she wouldn't wear it. We were doing all this emotional trauma for this nicer posture, which she didn't even care about. So we just let it go."

But back braces administered to scoliosis patients are anything but mere posture correction. Back braces are meant to slow or halt the progression of a child's scoliosis to avoid surgery and long-term pain or deformity. But though she had worn a back brace during high school,

Denise was completely unaware of this. Her spine's curvature had stopped when she had stopped growing; therefore, surgery was never even an option for her. She thought that, inevitably, the same would be true for her daughter. Denise was wrong.

"Before you knew it," she said, with traces of pain evident in her big brown eyes, "Erika started to complain of back pain, and it just came back to me—'Let me see your back.' It was a mess."

For five years, Erika's scoliosis had progressed freely and rapidly. Erika had refused to wear the brace; Denise had refused to make her daughter wear the brace. Erika led her life as if she didn't have scoliosis. By the age of fourteen, she was no longer the little girl who had worn a back brace. Her scoliosis had progressed considerably.

"I made an appointment again," Denise said. "Everyone just said, 'We're sorry to inform you, and we hate to see that it's progressed to this point, but she needs a spinal fusion.' Erika's curves now measured fifty degrees in the thoracic region and sixty-five degrees in the lumbar. . . . It took me two years of going through doctors and researching. I had to know that this was the last resort. It took me kind of a long time to accept it and that we had to do it."

Erika's curves continued their progression. In August 1997, her thoracic measurement was sixty degrees, her lumbar seventy-four degrees. Not only had the lateral curvature progressed, but rotation of the spine had begun to occur. Surgery was necessary immediately. In fact, Erika's spine was beyond the point at which doctors recommend surgery; in other words, she should have had the surgery sooner.

Both Erika and Denise will always wonder about the five years during which they were in denial about Erika's scoliosis. Would wearing the brace have prevented the surgery? Would Erika's emotional state after having been forced to wear the brace be worth a straight spine? But Erika and Denise know that they will never find answers to these questions.

"I, having been through a childhood with scoliosis, was still totally unaware of what could happen," Denise says. "If I had been more influenced or if there was more out there about it or even if the hospital had said something . . . who knows?"

SABINA

Upon meeting thirteen-year-old Sabina, I was captivated by her bubbly demeanor, her witty comments, and her confident poise. The blue "save the whales" t-shirt she was wearing, covered in part by her long,

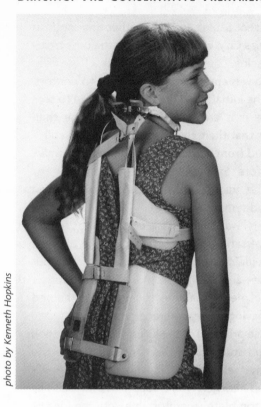

photo by Kenneth Hopkins

blonde locks, was the same color as her sparkling eyes.

"Do you like whales?" I asked.

"I'm an animal lover and a plant lover," she answered. "I'd like to be a botanist and a veterinarian when I grow up," she said.

As she spoke, her already vast knowledge of plants and animals became evident. Impressed by her apparent ambition to study the things she loves, I asked her how she had learned so much. Amidst her commitments to friends, homework, school dances, basketball, volleyball, softball, and swimming, she told me, were responsibilities as a volunteer at the Hutchinson County Zoo.

Bright, outgoing, and spirited in her pursuits, this adolescent exemplifies determination, optimism, and altruism. Hearing of her lifestyle and her accomplishments, one would not guess that Sabina has any problems; looking at her, however, one sees that something is wrong. Sabina's chin rests on a metal chin piece that is connected to her Milwaukee back brace. The metal brace extends from her chin to her hips, forcing her small body into a rigid, upright position and creating awkward bumps beneath the surface of her t-shirt so that the whale looks somewhat distorted.

Sabina's bout with scoliosis began over two years ago when the nurse at her school gave the students their annual physical examinations. The nurse detected Sabina's scoliosis and alerted Sabina's mother to the problem. At a visit to the pediatrician following the school nurse's diagnosis, X rays indicated to Sabina and her disbelieving mother that Sabina's spine had a forty-four-degree curve in the thoracic region. The pediatrician then sent Sabina and her mother to a scoliosis specialist at a hospital in Kansas City, who decided that the best treatment for Sabina would be bracing.

During the time that Sabina was absent from school due to doctors' visits, the school nurse took the initiative to orient the children to scoliosis; she taught them what it is and how it is treated. She then explained to the fifth graders that their classmate, Sabina, had scoliosis and that, when she returned from her absence, she would be wearing a back brace. Even before Sabina's return, the potential for ignorance and ridicule in the minds of her classmates had been replaced by understanding and sympathy.

Now that the word "scoliosis" was circulating around Sabina's school system, Sabina found, in conversation, that a certain junior in the high school had scoliosis too. The junior, named Jamie, was a smart, popular girl and an amazing athlete—and she had worn a back brace for six years! Jamie immediately became Sabina's mentor; she really helped Sabina adjust to the idea of having to wear a brace.

"Jamie and her father, the vice principal of the junior high school, took Sabina out for hamburgers and stuff during the transition, before the summer started," Sabina's mother remembers. "They were very helpful."

Though friends, family, and teachers were supportive of Sabina's condition, Sabina still wasn't completely comfortable with the idea of her scoliosis and her brace by the time her eleventh birthday arrived in June. Following a suggestion from her doctor, Sabina decided to have a "brace party" instead of a normal birthday party.

"We didn't say anything to the kids about what to bring," Sabina's mother recalls. "And they ended up bringing presents like body massage cream and body pillows . . . it was great. Then, during the four hours when Sabina could take the brace off, all the girls wanted to try it on. They all went into the bedroom—they were in there forever—and tried the brace on. That broke the ice for the kids; after that, nobody ever teased her."

"And at the party," added Sabina with a smile, "I named my brace. I call him Herby."

At this point, although Sabina's peers understood her condition, some other people didn't. But Sabina was finally confident enough about her brace and her scoliosis that potentially embarrassing inquiries became humorous to her.

"The little kids in my Mom's kindergarten class would stare," Sabina says. "They asked a lot of questions; they wanted to feel the brace and touch it. Some asked me if I had been in a car accident! Sometimes it was easier to just say 'yes' than to explain scoliosis to them."

"At the school dances, when Sabina would take her brace off for four hours, the boys who danced with her would exclaim, 'Whoa! You're so thin!'" Sabina's mother said, laughing.

"Yeah," Sabina added, "I'm so fat-looking with it [the brace]. And without it—a toothpick."

The boys in Sabina's class, however, are very accepting of her scoliosis. And the girls, sometimes to Sabina's dismay, are more understanding yet.

"There are a lot of girls who feel sorry for me," she says. "They get things for me and stuff; it drives me crazy. I don't like to be babied."

Despite the sympathy of her friends and teachers, Sabina has found that the outside world often isn't as understanding or nurturing as a school environment.

In January of Sabina's sixth-grade year, she returned to Kansas City for a check-up. The new X rays, taken at the checkup, showed that the brace was working, but minimally.

"Initially, when Sabina was X-rayed in her brace," Sabina's mother says, "the curve went down to thirty-seven degrees. At the January checkup, it went down to thirty-five degrees. Sabina's doctor was not a happy camper. He said to us that he hadn't yet ruled out surgery."

Three months later, however, the possibility of surgery seemed light years away. At Sabina's April checkup, her doctor found that her curve had decreased to twenty-eight degrees! Both doctor and patient were ecstatic. Sabina viewed her progress as a reason to keep wearing her brace and, as a result of Sabina's faithful brace-wearing, her curvature has gradually decreased even more.

"This one doctor was going to put rods in, and then we went to Sabina's doctor. He said that we should give Sabina as much growth (in the brace) as possible before surgery. The rods are the final and last resort," Sabina's mother says. So, until she stops growing and the brace is no longer effective, Sabina plans to ward off surgery by wearing her brace and staying active.

Though being active while wearing a back brace is a difficult task, Sabina is barely challenged by it. Doing the yoga "cat stretch," swimming laps, and participating in many other physical activities maintain Sabina's health and flexibility.

"Last year, my class had to run several laps around the gym for gym class," Sabina remembers. "I came in second—with the brace on. I beat almost everyone even though I was like ten times hotter than everyone else." Anyone who has ever worn a back brace knows of the heat that Sabina refers to; the brace seems to act like an insulator.

"Now that my spine's straighter, though, I have some neck pain. Actually, there's a very small curve in my neck," Sabina says. But Sabina's doctor has told her not to worry, for the neck curve and its implications are minimal. For now, Sabina will continue to wear the brace and visit her doctor every three months. She has become a full-fledged, devoted brace-wearer because she knows that she is still growing, and she will never back down and allow her scoliosis to increase.

Sabina could have used her brace as a reason to give up all physical activities, social events, and community service commitments. But Sabina is determined to live life as if she doesn't have scoliosis.

"Both my pediatrician and my scoliosis doctor said to me that nobody has a perfect body; everybody has to live with something. Even if you look at the wonderful models in these magazines, even though they look gorgeous, they have to live with some other defect. Nobody's perfect! And I think that whatever defect you have, you must learn to live with it."

And Sabina will do just that. She will continue to volunteer at the Hutchinson County Zoo, to study plants and animals, attend school dances, and do well in the races. In the midst of Sabina's busy life, her scoliosis—along with Herby—fades into the periphery.

JENNIFER

Jen was an active jazz and tap dancer, a skilled softball and basketball player, and a devoted gymnast when, at the age of ten, she found out that she had juvenile idiopathic scoliosis. The prescribed treatment for Jen's scoliosis was wearing a back brace for twenty-three hours every day. Agreeable, Jen decided that she would wear the brace for as long as she needed to so that she could solve the problem that her doctors called "scoliosis" and get on with her life.

"Jen really adjusted well to it," her mother, Jane, remembers. "She was determined to wear the brace faithfully and to just get this [her scoliosis] over with."

Perhaps Jen's determination was fostered by the fact that her orthopedic doctor told her that she would have to wear her brace for a definite period of two years.

"Even in her hour without it, she kept it on," Jane says. "She was really, really good about it for two whole years."

For two years, Jen wore the same back brace faithfully. Over the course of those years, she visited her orthotist every six months for X rays and examinations. The orthotist chose to alternate taking Jen's X rays with her brace on and off. Toward the end of the two-year period, the orthotist informed Jen and her mother that Jen's curve had increased from its original twenty-eight degrees to about thirty degrees as Jen had grown. Both Jen and her mother knew that any progression in Jen's scoliosis curve was likely the result of a recent slacking in brace wear. As Jen had started to make the transition from childhood to her teens, she also discovered her doctor's "two-year" promise was incorrect. She then found brace-wearing to be a lot more difficult.

"I'd say maybe in the third year with her brace, Jen started developing a little, and she started to get uncomfortable," recalls Jane.

"I wouldn't wear it to school," Jen admits. "The only time I wore it was when I got home from school."

"Sometimes I'd leave for work before Jen left for school in the morning," Jane says. "When I would come home in the middle of the day for lunch, I'd find Jen's brace on her bed."

"In fourth grade, when I first got the brace, I didn't mind it. All the kids at school thought it was cool and stuff," says Jen. "But then I started to get sick of it. By sixth grade—the last year of grammar school, I wasn't really wearing it anymore. And I was *not* going to wear it in middle school."

At their next visit to Jen's doctor, Jen and her mother hesitated to talk about the fact that Jen had stopped wearing her brace for the prescribed number of hours.

"Our appointment with the doctor was coming up in October," Jane remembers. "We couldn't even try to squeeze Jen into it until the appointment. She had grown out of it, but we hadn't even realized it because she hadn't been wearing it. So we just carried it to the doctor's office with us. The brace was lying on the floor of the office."

"The doctor indicated that all of Jen's hard work [wearing the brace for two years] had been in vain just because she hadn't worn it as much as she should have for the past two or three months. He actually compared her to someone who had been running for a field goal (a touchdown) and had fumbled at the last five yards." Naturally, Jen was upset by her doctor's comments.

Jen had started middle school—without her brace—that September. After her traumatic October doctor's visit, she didn't want to think about her scoliosis until the new year arrived. Jen's mother did not know what to do. She could not bear to ignore Jen's scoliosis; she knew that would be the worst thing to do. So she took Jen back to the doctor and was told that Jen would have to wear a brace for at least another eighteen months.

"I talked to her, and she said, 'I'm not getting another brace!' I said that she had to. At this point, we just had to," says Jane. To Jen's dismay, she and her mother soon returned to the orthotist and had Jen fitted for her second brace.

"Boy, was she miserable," says Jane. "The new brace was twice the size of the other one because her upper curve had gotten so bad that the orthotist put extra padding there and made the brace go higher."

"I wore it for a month—not even—and then I decided that was it," Jen says. "I can't wear it again." A few weeks after Jen had stopped wearing her second brace, Jane decided, once again, to take action. She contacted a different orthopedic surgeon and made an appointment for Jen.

Jen's new orthopedic surgeon patiently took the time to explain everything—her condition and all of her treatment options. The doctor discussed the consequences of her wearing the brace and the consequences of her not wearing the brace; he also informed her that her scoliosis had about a fifty percent chance of progressing if she chose not to wear the brace. Regardless of what the doctor said, though, Jen maintained her stance on bracing. Jen felt both embittered and discouraged about bracing. At the youthful age of thirteen, she made the very serious and difficult decision not to wear a back brace anymore. She would take the chance of allowing her scoliosis to progress. A short time after she had made this decision, Jen, at fifteen, would be forced to come to terms with it.

ANTHONY

In September of 1994, Anthony was busy being a high school sophomore and playing on the varsity soccer team. His world consisted of school, soccer, and friends, and his horizons reached as far as the hockey and lacrosse seasons that lay ahead. When Anthony walked into his doctor's office for his back-to-school physical that year, his mind was elsewhere and his thoughts were consumed by the details of his fifteen-year-old life. When Anthony left that office, his mind was shocked; his thoughts were consumed by his diagnosis with adolescent idiopathic scoliosis.

Suspecting that Anthony's newfound scoliosis would require the attention of a specialist, Anthony's pediatrician sent him to an ortho-pedic doctor for evaluation. In turn, the orthopedic doctor, whom Anthony saw that October, referred him to a pediatric orthopedic spe-cialist. X rays showed that Anthony had a twenty-eight-degree curve in the thoracic region of his spine, spanning from the T5 vertebra to the T12 vertebra. And at the time of his diagnosis, Anthony was only a Risser 0; in other words, he had a lot of growing time remaining and was on the threshold of the period during which his scoliosis would increase most rapidly and dramatically.

Because of Anthony's preference to forego brace-wearing during the school day and his commitment to his busy after-school sports sched-ule, his doctor decided that a Charleston bending brace would be the best treatment for Anthony. In January of 1995, after Anthony had been wearing his back brace every night for three months, he returned to his orthopedist for a checkup. At this followup visit, Anthony's doctor detected a 1.5-centimeter high rib prominence in the right thoracic region of Anthony's back, as well as an elevation of his right shoulder

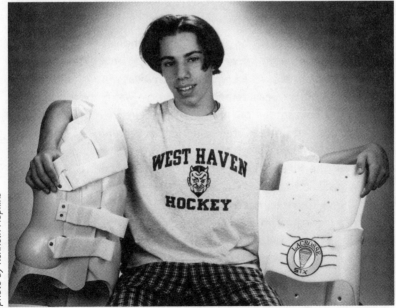

photo by Kenneth Hopkins

and a protrusion of his shoulder blade. New X rays showed that Anthony was now a Risser 1; he was one step further toward skeletal maturity but still had a lot of growing to do. Despite wearing the Charleston brace, Anthony had not stopped his curve from progressing. In just three months, the curve that had previously measured twenty-eight degrees now measured thirty-five degrees. Concerned about the progression of Anthony's curve, his doctor advised him to continue wearing the Charleston brace and return for another checkup in two months. Though adolescent scoliosis patients do not normally visit their doctors as frequently as every two months, Anthony's doctor knew that his curve was progressing quickly and felt that he required close observation.

Anthony's March 1995 X ray showed that his curve had progressed from thirty-five to thirty-eight degrees. In June 1995, Anthony's curve had progressed to forty-three degrees. The Charleston brace was not working. In an attempt to halt the progression of Anthony's stubborn curve, his doctor prescribed full-time brace wear for Anthony; he suggested getting a Boston brace to wear during the day and keeping the Charleston brace for nighttime wear.[9]

"At this point, we were told that his [Anthony's] curve was very difficult to control and that even full-time Boston brace wear might fail," remembers Anthony's mother, Pat. "If that was the case, the doctor said he would recommend surgery once Anthony's curve had exceeded fifty degrees."

In September 1995, X rays taken while Anthony was in his Boston brace illustrated that the curve measured an apparent (not actual) thirty-four degrees. X rays taken while Anthony was *not* in the brace disclosed that the true measurement of his curve was forty-four degrees. Anthony, his doctor, and his parents were elated to find the Boston brace had been effective in stabilizing Anthony's curve over the course of the summer. Once school began, however, Anthony's commitment to wearing the Boston brace during the day waned. Now a junior, Anthony disliked having to wear the brace at school and was unable to wear it during sports games and practices. As a result of this slacking in daytime brace wear, Anthony's curve progressed three more degrees by December 1995. And, despite his doctor's advice to continue wearing his two braces and warnings about the possibility of surgery, sixteen-year-old Anthony did not want to acknowledge that any treatment was necessary; he continued to wear his Charleston brace at night, but he only wore his Boston brace at select times of his choosing.

"Anthony did not want to hear the word 'surgery' or the news that he had to wear the brace twenty-two to twenty-three hours a day," Pat recalls. "He was so focused on his soccer, hockey, and lacrosse, and he was not about to let his scoliosis get in the way of his sports."

By June 1996, the lacrosse season was almost over and Anthony was completing his junior year in high school. Since Anthony's last visit to the hospital, his orthopedist had moved from Connecticut to North Carolina, and his position at the hospital had been filled by a new doctor. After examining his case and history, the new doctor advised Anthony to stop wearing the back braces. Anthony's curve now measured forty-six degrees, and—perhaps due to the fact that Anthony was nearly finished growing or the reality of his unwillingness to *fully* comply with brace wear—the braces were no longer affecting the curve's progression. Despite what his new doctor said, Anthony still wore the Charleston brace during the night. Anthony's decision to wear his brace even after he was told that he didn't need to is not uncommon among adolescents in braces. Because of the temporary back comfort a brace can give by taking pressure off muscles, or because of mere habit, many people continue to wear their braces for progressively shorter periods of time after they have been told that they no longer need to wear the braces.

Therefore, following a summer of wearing his Charleston brace at night, Anthony, along with his parents, was not surprised when told that his curve had progressed to fifty-two degrees. At this point, Anthony's doctor made a strong recommendation that Anthony have surgery. Though the need for surgery was not immediate, it was necessary; there was no other treatment option for Anthony's scoliosis.

"Anthony was devastated," says Pat. Eventually, though, Anthony came to terms with his scoliosis and with the fact that he was facing surgery. Time played an enormous factor in this attitude change. Over time, Anthony matured and came to view his situation in a different light. He would have surgery just two and a half years after he had been diagnosed; he would approach his surgery with an attitude marked by thorough acceptance, complete confidence, and a cool composure; and he would be dancing all night at his senior prom just two weeks after his spine had been fused. What a guy!

TIPS ON BRACE WEAR

CLOTHING

The good news is that you will need a new wardrobe (or at least new pants and skirts)! Unfortunately, I had already completed my back-to-school shopping when I found out that I needed to wear a brace. I put those clothes aside to wear at special times or during the six hours I didn't have to wear a brace (my doctor prescribed eighteen hours of brace wear). The day I received my brace, we went out to lunch and clothes shopping—with my brace on! It was quite humorous as my mother and I picked out clothes that would camouflage my brace. I wore pants that were a size bigger in order to fit comfortably over my hips, which were now covered with my brace. Fortunately, baggy clothes were "in." No problem there! I wore large longsleeve t-shirts and/or large flannel shirts. I favored overalls, which really were perfect. One problem was that my shirts eventually wore out in the same place, where the brace ended in my upper back region. I learned not to wear expensive clothes to school! Then I would balance my heroic brace-wearing with an occasional short skirt and tiny fitted t-shirt or a fitted dress when I didn't need to wear my brace or when I was going somewhere special. At the end of my brace-wearing year, I remember the reaction of my classmates when they saw me in a bathing suit at a school pool party! That's the fun part—revealing who you really are under the brace!

COMFORT MEASURES

Wearing plastic on your entire torso makes you so hot! I didn't wear a coat the entire winter and still, oftentimes, my t-shirt would be soaking wet. If you're not comfortable, you won't wear the brace—so it's best to be comfortable!

◆ Wear a one hundred percent cotton undershirt under your brace. Never wear the brace directly on your skin. The undershirt absorbs perspiration, prevents odor, preserves the integrity of your skin, and helps to maintain the good condition of your brace.

◆ Maintain good body hygiene. Bathe daily.

◆ Be alert to reddened or irritated areas. While discoloration of the skin from brace-wearing is usually not anything to worry about, you don't want any part of your skin breaking down. Alert your orthotist; perhaps your brace was tightened too much or is putting pressure in the wrong areas.

◆ Creams and lotions are not recommended, since softening of the skin could promote breakdown. I do recommend Gold Bond Powder or another body powder for irritated areas.

◆ Be faithful to your orthotist appointments. They may be every four to six weeks. Your brace, much like the braces you wear on your teeth, needs to be tightened to be effective. While this will not be the most comfortable for a day or two, take advantage of the appointment to ask questions and have your orthotist "look things over."

TIPS FOR SUMMER BRACE WEAR

Your family and friends need to appreciate how warm it can be for you at this time of the year. When underarm rubbing was no longer an issue for me, I oftentimes resorted to camisole wear with shorts and just put the brace over everything.

◆ Stay in air conditioning as much as possible.

◆ Try to busy yourself with indoor activities that will provide you with an air-conditioned environment.

◆ Careful when you go to the beach without your brace! You don't need a sunburn.

ACTIVITIES

You are just wearing a brace! You don't have anything wrong with you that dictates physical limitations. Talk to your doctor about what you should and should not do. Generally, contact sports should be avoided and, of course, gymnastics. But you can enjoy these activities during your time out of the brace.

How to Take Care of Your Brace

When you receive your brace, it is like a new car—spanking clean. After months of wear, it gradually becomes discolored and not so clean. You can clean your brace with a damp, soapy cloth as often as you like. It helps to keep your brace clean and helps you to feel fresh.

Tips for Sleeping

Let's face it, who will ever admit to comfortable sleeping with a brace? I will say that although it took me a while to get used to it, I did sleep with it with no problem.

Use lots of pillows for support in front and in back, and in between your legs for side sleeping. Look for specialty catalogs or stores, such as Relax the Back, which provide comfort measures such as special pillows and mattresses, if you deem them necessary.

BRACE WEARING 101

For the Teenage Brace Wearer

◆ Know *why* you are wearing the brace. Get as much information as you can about how bracing can stop the progression of your curve. Know about the different kinds of braces, and why your doctor suggests the kind that's right for you. Ask your doctor and orthotist all the questions you need to ask. Knowing about scoliosis and why you are wearing the brace may help make the process of wearing it easier for you. This is *your* body and *your* future that is at stake. Take an active role in your own treatment.

◆ Make sure that your brace is as comfortable as possible. Know that your body will need some time to get used to the brace. Just like an athlete who begins a new exercise plan, you may feel muscle aches and pains in the first few weeks of brace-wear. This is normal; don't get discouraged. Your body is using muscles differently than the way you are used to using them. You are also going through a physical and emotional training; time will help you here. Sleeping may be difficult at first, but do not break down and remove the brace in the middle of the night. In getting used to wearing a brace, persistence is key. If you are experiencing skin irritation, chafing, or undue discomfort, call your doctor or orthotist. Simple bracing adjustments can make all the difference in how you feel.

◆ Take things one step at a time. Don't start planning the rest of your life around brace wear and scoliosis! Do it a day at a time, a week at a time. Deal with each issue as it arises. Imagine, if on the first day of high school, you had to think and plan for every test you had to take in the next four years, who you might go with to the senior prom, what you might major in when you get into the college you choose, and so on. If you think this way, you may never put your foot through the front door of your school and take that first step! The same goes with brace wear. Deal with situations one at a time. Don't overwhelm yourself by trying to solve every possible issue you think might arise.

◆ I know that it can be difficult to find others in your situation, and difficulty finding people with whom you can relate can only worsen preexisting feelings of being alone and "different." I also know that you do not feel like going to some support group meeting and announcing, "Hello, my name is so and so, and I have scoliosis." Even though *you* may have scoliosis, you may conclude that you are still unlike the people who seek support for scoliosis. After all, despite the brace you're wearing, you are a "normal" person—not one of those people who needs the help of others, right? Wrong. I cannot emphasize enough how finding other people close to your age who are wearing or who have already worn a brace can help you to feel more comfortable with your own scoliosis and back brace. Finding people who can identify with your situation can make you feel a lot better about having scoliosis—even if you weren't feeling that bad to begin with. Your doctor can direct you to other patients or to self-help groups with adolescent members. Meet with other people (maybe by phone, letter, or on-line) who have "been there" and "done that." Find out what these people's brace-wearing experiences were like and how they managed different situations. Take charge! The more people you know who are wearing or who have worn a brace, the broader your support network will be. Before you know it, you will be the one encouraging and answering questions for those who are just starting out.

◆ Humor, humor, humor! Life isn't all about seriousness; even things that have the potential to be grave can actually be funny. This brace isn't sacred or above reproach! If you can find things to laugh about or joke about regarding brace wear, do it! People with a sense of humor—those who can see the lighter side of life's curves—cope better and feel better about themselves and their circumstances. Humor can diffuse a lot of stress and tension. It can put things in a whole new perspective. So, in dealing with your brace, use humor whenever you can!

◆ Wear clothes that are a size or two larger than those you would usually wear. This will give you an easier time in daily movement. It will also make the brace less noticeable and will preserve your old clothes from the wear and tear that braces can cause.

◆ We personalize our wardrobes, our possessions, and ourselves. Why not, then, personalize our braces? Consider decorating your brace to suit your personal style. We've seen people use colors or symbols or ornaments on their braces to express their individuality, styles, and tastes. If this idea appeals to you, why not "go for it?" You can be as creative with this as fashion designers are with external, more public garments and gear. Who knows? You might start a trend that ends up on next year's Paris fashion runway!

◆ Think ahead about how you'd like to handle questions about your brace. Always remember this rule of thumb: People take their cues on how to react to your brace from *you*. The more confident and less defensive you appear, the better, but do not try to act like someone other than yourself; your answers to questions concerning your brace should suit your personality. Your answers to people's questions can be as short, lengthy, personal, or objective as you want them to be. They can be factual or medical for those who do not wish to talk about the feelings they have concerning their brace. Some scoliosis patients like to create fantastic and creative stories to answer people's questions. Again, consider using humor. You might want to role-play your answers with parents, brothers or sisters, or supportive peers. That way, you'll get some feedback. If this doesn't suit you, practice by yourself in front of a mirror. Try to have some fun with this. Good answers on your part can go a long way toward normalizing a potentially uncomfortable or awkward situation. Some people's questions or statements may sound offensive; others may just sound dumb. Whatever the case, just remember to keep your cool, your poise, and your control. Your answers will come more easily as you become more used to people asking you questions over time.

FOR PARENTS OF A BRACE WEARER

It is important to remember that compliance with brace treatment is in no way an immediate, here-and-now, pleasurable experience for your child. All rewards for it lie somewhere in the future. By contrast, there are often immediate rewards for non-compliance with few immediate negative consequences. As such, your child may be coping with some strong conflicting feelings about brace wear, many of which push toward non-adherence. How can you encourage your child to wear the brace? The following are some suggestions.

◆ Be well-informed about the role of bracing in the general management of scoliosis. Ask your doctor any and all questions you may have. You can educate yourself by reading current books and articles on scoliosis and by going on-line. You can also join local chapters of national support groups. This will put you in direct contact with other parents facing similar issues and will give you first-hand information about how other families handle a variety of brace-wear topics. Many self-help chapters have regular presentations by physicians and allied health professionals with up-to-date information for you. National organizations have regular publications to which you can subscribe. Being well-informed will give you the long-range viewpoint you need to encourage your child's brace-wear compliance.

◆ Communicate with your child. Find a time and a place to talk regularly, even if only for ten minutes. Be an active listener. Ask questions, respond, look at your child. Talk about everything, not just brace wear. Remember names of friends, teachers, and the previous day's concerns. Your child will feel important if you remember what is important to him or her. Even if your teen doesn't demand your attention, he or she still needs it.

Try not only to listen to the words your child speaks, but to the feelings underneath the words. Pay attention to tone of voice and body posture. Is your child happy or excited, or disappointed or rejected? Look for cues that communicate the feelings. They are a vital part of most communications. Losing touch with feelings, denying their existence, repressing them, or even ridiculing them can only diminish self-esteem. In talking with your child or teen, you are developing your relationship with him or her. This, in turn, will strengthen your child, and inner strength is a necessity for those facing life's challenges. It is most important when facing the emotional strains that can result from wearing a brace over time through the already bumpy road of adolescence.

◆ Share concerns with your spouse; talk with your partner. Privately, discuss your feelings with each other. Acknowledge these feelings—frustrations, worries, fears, disappointments, and so on. Recognize any differences that might exist. Then, be sure that you are "on the same wavelength" in supporting your child's efforts. Even if you have different communication styles, your message to your child about brace wearing should be consistent. Try not to let possible differences or disagreements in other areas of your marriage get in the way here. Your child will respond to ambivalent or mixed messages about the importance of wearing the brace with his or her own mixed feelings and behaviors. This is a sure recipe for noncompliance—something you want to avoid. Try to be consistent in supporting and understanding each other. This is the best thing you can do at this time for your child and your family.

◆ Where possible, involve siblings and other family members in supporting the cause. Help brothers and sisters to recognize their role in supporting their sibling's treatment efforts. Involving them may help them overcome their perceptions that an inordinate amount of attention is being given to the brace wearer. Such perceptions could result in a certain amount of jealousy, which might sabotage the cause. Grandparents and aunts and uncles can also voice their support and best wishes in their own style. They will need to take their cues from the information provided to them in a factual, level-headed manner by parents.

◆ Recognize the partnership among the physician, patient, and family. Treatment professionals must remind themselves that bracing can be especially difficult for teenagers. They need to communicate their support in a warm and empathetic manner. Professionals and parents must help the patient to perceive himself or herself as a prime mover in a treatment plan that can prevent the development of more serious problems. The patient must perceive himself or herself as making a real difference in his or her own health and well-being. Patients need praise for their efforts, compliance, and accomplishments in their daily work; this periodic praise should continue for the duration of the patient's time in the brace. If you are treated at a scoliosis clinic, it is most helpful for you to see one particular doctor with consistency so that you get to know him or her, so that he or she gets to know you, and so that you can hear praise and encouragement from that one, significant provider— and not any random doctor with whom you happen to be paired.

DEALING WITH NONCOMPLIANCE

If your child will not wear the brace for the prescribed length of time, or if you are at a complete impasse regarding bracewear, consider the following:

◆ Keep communication open. Avoid arguments; they only make matters worse.

◆ Try to understand the reason for the child's or teenager's not wanting to wear the brace. Different reasons require different solutions.

"This thing hurts," "My boyfriend doesn't like it," and "Kids at school make fun of me" need to be addressed differently.

◆ Look for things in common with your opposing viewpoints. For example, you both want a healthy outcome; you both want to avoid surgery—you just have differing paths to these ends. Try to negotiate and compromise your opposing viewpoints; the result will be a faster route to your desired ends.

◆ Participate in local support group chapters. You may get a fresh perspective and trade ideas with other parents who have been in a similar situation. Keep yourself informed about scoliosis and developments in the field.

◆ Try to involve your child in support groups with teen members. If your child can talk to someone (preferably someone similar in age) who knows exactly what he or she is going through and who can fully relate, your child will have found an invaluble resource for comfort, encouragement, recognition, and helpful tips.

◆ Explore the range of bracing options with your orthotist.

◆ Explore the possibility of a time-out from brace wear with your doctor. Also, ask if the brace can be removed during specific activities.

◆ If your child completely refuses to wear the brace, and if you feel as though you have tried everything, do not lose faith in or respect for your child. A child or teenager is not a bad or weak person because he or she refuses to wear a brace; perhaps he or she just can't do it. Don't belittle your child or the difficulty; this will only hurt self-esteem. Always keep the negotiation door open. Many things (including attitudes toward bracing) can change in adolescence with the passage of time.

BRACING FOR EFFECTIVE TREATMENT

- Children with curves ranging from twenty to forty degrees
- Teenagers who have at least a few months of skeletal growth remaining, with curves ranging from twenty to forty degrees

BRACING FOR COMFORT
(AND NOT NECESSARILY EFFECTIVENESS)

- Children and teenagers, perhaps with back pain, whose curves exceed forty degrees
- Adults with back pain and poor posture related to scoliotic curves

POOR CANDIDATES FOR BRACING

- People who wish to *correct* (and not just to halt) their scoliosis curves, usually large curves of more than forty-five to fifty degrees in the immature patient
- People who are considerably overweight
- Patients with thoracic lordosis (swayback) in association with scoliosis; *i.e.*, lordosis loss

THE FUNDAMENTALS OF BRACING

- To halt progression of curve(s)
- Compliance with prescribed number of hours of brace wearing is essential for achieving success

CHAPTER 3

Scoliosis Heroes

I f you have been diagnosed with scoliosis, you know that a flood of feelings ranging from sorrow to anger is bound to accompany such a diagnosis. Feelings of unhappiness that inevitably accompany any scoliosis diagnosis can only be amplified if your scoliosis and the treatment it requires promise to prohibit you from pursuing a sport or activity you love. In a situation where a favorite sport or activity is threatened by the prospect of bracing or surgery, some people give up their activities and allow their scoliosis to defeat them; others continue with their favorite activities, all the while ignoring their scoliosis and allowing it to become more severe as time passes.

The following people are heroes and heroines who have adeptly combined treating their scoliosis with excelling in their favorite sports and activities. Despite their scoliosis, these people have devotedly pursued particular activities and areas of interest; and, despite their involvement with these activities and areas of interest, they have not lost sight of the acute importance of treating their scoliosis. Some of these people have had to wear back braces; some have had to undergo surgery. Whatever the case, throughout their respective struggles with scoliosis, all have demonstrated immense courage and have remained committed to pursuing their passions and dreams. Though they are relatively young, they are masters at keeping calm and cool while they combine scoliosis with life. And though they are all humble when it comes to discussing their achievements, they are a tremendous inspiration to us all.

JAMES BLAKE

Tennis Champion

When James was just three years old, his parents took him to the Armory at the corner of 142nd Street and Fifth Avenue in his native New York City. It was there that James picked up his first tennis ball, gripped his first racquet, and got his first taste of the game that would come to shape his life. When James was five years old, his family moved from New York to Connecticut, where James continued to play tennis. And when James was fifteen years old, his mother took him to his pediatrician's office. It was there that he was diagnosed with scoliosis, referred to an orthopedic doctor, and threatened by the prospect of a constraint on his budding tennis career.

James was a freshman in high school when his pediatrician detected the curvature in his spine. At first, the pediatrician noticed James's scoliosis but failed to mention anything about it to James and his mother because he found the curvature so obvious that he assumed something was already being done about it. Later in the examination, James's pediatrician inquired about the treatment being used to halt the progression of his scoliotic curve. James and his mother looked at the doctor with bewildered expressions; the doctor knew then that, while James's scoliosis had been obvious to *him*, it had not been obvious to James and his family. The pediatrician explained scoliosis to James and his mother and that the appropriate treatment for James, at that point, would probably be bracing.

Upon discussing his diagnosis with his family members, fifteen-year-old James found out that the scoliosis was a trait he had inherited from his father's side of the family. James's stepbrother on his father's side, who also happened to play tennis, had scoliosis, too. James's father had noticed the deformity in James's stepbrother when he had seen him bending over one day. James's stepbrother ended up being formally diagnosed with a thirty-degree scoliotic curve and being braced for a

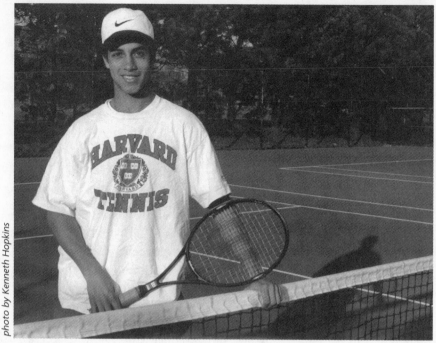

photo by Kenneth Hopkins

James on the outdoor courts at Harvard

few years until he reached skeletal maturity. Interestingly, James's full brother, Thomas Jr., never exhibited any trace of scoliosis. The incidence of scoliosis in James's extended family just goes to show that inheritance of the trait occurs at random.

Shortly after he had been diagnosed by his pediatrician, James visited the orthopedic surgeon to whom he had been referred by his pediatrician. James's X rays showed that he had a thoracic curve measuring twenty-nine degrees; his diagnostic tests showed that he had a few years left before he would reach skeletal maturity. The orthopedic surgeon determined that the appropriate treatment for James would be bracing—just as the pediatrician had expected. He told James that he would have to wear this back brace for eighteen hours every day.

Two questions arose in James's mind. One, what effect would his scoliosis have on his playing tennis? And two, would his parents be able to finance his back brace (which would cost almost $2,000) and his periodic checkups? As it turned out, James practiced tennis during the short time each day that he did not have to be in his brace. And his parents found out about the Shriners' Hospital for Crippled Children[10]—a hospital that selects its patients carefully and then pays for their care.

James and his family visited the Shriners' Hospital in Massachusetts. James describes the doctors there as being "incredibly nice" and the treatment as being "completely free." The Shriners' Hospital immediately provided James with a back brace and scheduled him for checkups every four months over the next several years. Over the course of those years, James grew considerably and went through not one, but *three* braces, all of which were paid for by Shriners. In the meantime, James allowed nothing to stand in his way from achieving his goal in tennis.

Throughout his years in high school, James devoted most—if not all—of his free time to improving his tennis game. James did not make tennis his hobby or his sport; he made it his life. During the same years that he was wearing his brace, he ascended national tennis rankings to become the number one player in the country for the eighteen-and-under division when he was just seventeen.

At every tennis practice and tournament James attended throughout his high school years, he could always be seen carrying not one but two tennis bags. In one bag he carried his racquet and other tennis equipment; in the other bag he carried his back brace. Though wearing the brace for eighteen hours each day proved to be somewhat of a hassle to someone who spent most of his time training on the tennis courts, James was committed to wearing the brace as much as he was able. James's commitment to bringing his back brace everywhere he went and to wearing the cumbersome apparatus as frequently as he could was rooted in his apprehension of the possibility of his curve's progressing.

"They [doctors] have said if it [the scoliosis] gets much worse, they might have to fuse my back, and if that happened, I wouldn't be able to play competitive tennis again. That was scary," James says.[11]

Despite the omnipresent threat of having to undergo surgery and the onus of having to wear a back brace, James has kept his spirits high and his focus on the tennis court throughout his teenage years. He was the number one ranked tennis player in the boys eighteen-and-under division in the United States Tennis Association while in high school. James has played in international tennis tournaments, including the U.S. Open and the French Open. He worked hard in high school and earned a place at Harvard University. As a freshman at Harvard, he became the third ranked player in the national college tennis league. Never does he pity himself or consider his straight-spined opponents to have an advantage over him. James takes his scoliosis in stride, treats it cooperatively and quietly, and goes about achieving his goals in a determined yet serene fashion. James maintains that his periodic visits to the Shriners' Hospital have helped him to keep his scoliosis in perspective.

"It helps keep me positive, with my head up," he says. "I have to go to the hospital for crippled children, because scoliosis is crippling when it gets really bad. I get to see a lot of patients there. When I go in there, I am one of the few who actually walk in on their own. It's a good experience to help me realize how lucky I am just to be able to play tennis. And to be able to play at this level is just incredible."[12]

Presently, James has reached skeletal maturity. As he finishes his sophomore year at Harvard, he only wears his brace at night, for he is slowly weaning himself off brace wear. Occasionally, he visits a chiropractor for "adjustments" whenever his back "goes out." During the period when he wore his brace full-time, his scoliosis curve stabilized at about thirty degrees. Now that he is fully grown, James hopes that the curve in his spine has stopped progressing for good. Thus far, James's curve has shown no progression after he has reached skeletal maturity, and James has been free to travel around the country pursuing his tennis career. While his spine seems to be stable now, though, James always keeps in mind that, when it comes to scoliosis, anything can happen.

"I always try to stay optimistic," says James. "I just have a feeling I'm always going to be playing tennis. I just hope that I am."[13] It looks like he will be!

James's Current Tennis Standings

- Men's Singles Title at the Rolex International Championships—February 8, 1999 (the first Ivy League player to win this title since 1983).
- College playing is 20-1 as a sophomore, and 57-6 overall.
- ITA ranking—#1 in singles; #5 in doubles.
- Won first USTA Futures title—January 1999.
- USTA Boys 18-and-under National Championship—1997 finalist.
- USTA Clay Court and Indoor titles—First Place.

JEANETTE LEE

The Black Widow

A first-generation Korean American born into a bilingual household, Jeanette Lee was nurtured by a unique brand of the archetypal American ideal of opportunity—one seasoned with the richness of traditional Korean values. This coalescence of cultures and value systems with which Jeanette was raised served her well. As a young girl growing up in Brooklyn, New York, she demonstrated intelligence and determination that enabled her to stand out amongst her peers and to earn a place at the prestigious Bronx High School of Science. But before entering high school, she was forced to handle an obstacle that had never been a part of her American dream.

Like many teenage girls, Jeanette had been self-conscious about her body for some time and had avoided wearing revealing clothing or bathing suits. For this reason, even Jeanette's family had not seen what Jeanette remembers as being a "flat-chested and scrawny" figure. At thirteen, though, Jeanette was finally ready to embrace some

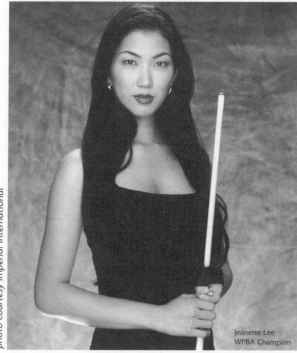

photo courtesy Imperial International

Jeanette Lee
WPBA Champion

self-confidence, to wear a bathing suit, and to cast away some of her early adolescent physical concerns. On a family outing to the beach one day, thirteen-year-old Jeanette sported a bikini— her first ever. Upon Jeanette's removal of her exterior clothing, her mother gasped at the appearance of her daughter's back. Jeanette's small torso was contorted by the severe "S" curve in her spine. No one had ever noticed this deformity because Jeanette had been so shy about her body and had kept it hidden so well. Jeanette's mother, a registered nurse, quickly recognized the problem with her daughter's spine and promptly took Jeanette to a series of doctors.

Within a matter of weeks, several doctors agreed that Jeanette's scoliosis was severe enough to warrant immediate surgery. Though Jeanette was relatively young and had not yet experienced her adolescent growth spurt, her primary scoliosis curve measured fifty-five degrees. Wearing a back brace would have limited results, so surgery was her best option—not only to correct her scoliosis, but to halt its rapid progression. Thus, at age thirteen, Jeanette underwent a spinal fusion with placement of Harrington rods. Prior to the surgery, Jeanette remembers being "really scared." She did not know how long the surgery would take, what it would entail, how quickly she would recover, or what she would look and feel like post-operatively. Terrified, Jeanette was wheeled into the operating room. The next thing she remembers is waking up after the surgery.

Not only was Jeanette unable to vocalize her discomfort, but she was unable to move; her entire body felt incredibly "sluggish and slow" under the influence of the sedatives in the post-operative period. To this day, Jeanette does not know how long she remained in the hospital after her surgery. Her sense of time was clouded by her post-operative discomfort. After Jeanette had regained her strength and returned home, she was bound for eight months in a post-surgical body cast and then in a back brace. After her surgery, Jeanette longed for someone to talk to, but she did not find anyone who could relate to her.

When Jeanette was eighteen, she discovered something that would alter her attitude, shift her focus off of her scoliosis, and change her life forever. One day, she saw an old man playing pool.

"I was just mesmerized by how beautiful the game was," she remembers. "Each time you break the balls, you create a new configuration . . . a new puzzle to solve. You create your own art."

Jeanette knew at that point that she wanted to learn to play pool. Almost immediately, she immersed herself in all facets of the game. Before she knew it, Jeanette was practicing pool for ten hours each day, reading books on pool, befriending old-time pool professionals, and exploring other billiard games. Along with her budding interest, though, came increased back pain.

"I probably started playing too much pool," Jeanette says. Being bent over all the time while playing the game created an incredible strain on the instrumentation in Jeanette's back. Yet Jeanette was not about to give up her newfound passion simply because her back hurt.

"For the first time in my life, I was able to focus on something other than my own unworthiness," she says. For years, Jeanette had viewed herself as being a worthless, deformed creature. Now, though, she had found a distinct talent; something that made her feel purposeful, exhilarated, and beautiful. Despite her chronic back pain, Jeanette continued to practice pool and to strive for excellence in her game. And, in a short time, her hard work began to pay off.

The intelligence and determination she had demonstrated since childhood empowered Jeanette to develop unparalleled skill in playing pool. Shortly after her emergence on the pool-playing scene, Jeanette received the nickname "The Black Widow" from her contemporaries in the world of billiards because of what has been called her "tenacious ability to devour opponents and her tendency to wear only black during competition."

Four years after she picked up her first cue, Jeanette turned professional and joined the Women's Professional Billiards Association Tour. Less than a year later, she had become one of the top ten pool players in the world and was runner-up in the world championships. One year after that, Jeanette became the number one ranked female pool player in the world, maintaining that ranking for two years. A strikingly beautiful woman who has taken the billiards world by storm and has glamorized the game of pool, Jeanette has traveled around the world and has become an internationally renowned figure. Her flawless appearance, superior ability in pool, and confident demeanor, though, belie the metal-laden spine that no one can see and the chronic pain that no one knows exists.

Throughout her career, Jeanette has had to deal with the unrelenting back pain wrought by her scoliosis and the Harrington rods that remain implanted inside her. She unfortunately developed pseudarthrosis (failed fusion) in the L3 and L4 vertebrae, has had a piece of her instrumentation come loose, and has needed periodic intervertebral injections of medicine for her pain. Many doctors have told her that she has two choices; she can either deal with the pain, or undergo corrective surgery during which her Harrington rods would be replaced by more modern instrumentation. Ultimately, Jeanette plans to have surgery in order to maintain her health and improve her quality of life. But she does not wish to have surgery until she has lived out her dream and finished her career.

In the meantime, Jeanette sees a doctor about her scoliosis every two to three months and depends on the intervertebral injections of pain medicine she often receives to alleviate some of her pain. She also swims, stretches, and exercises on a regular basis in order to keep in shape, maintain flexibility, and relieve some of the muscular pain in her back. While Jeanette values exercise and pain medication as means of helping her excel as a professional pool player despite her severe back pain, she hails her husband, billiards professional George Breedlove, as the most helpful agent of all. Jeanette describes George as "the best" and "most supportive" husband.

"God really blessed me with my husband," she says. "He's unbelievable."

Due to back pain, Jeanette is no longer able to practice pool for ten to twenty hours each day, as she has been known to do in the past. She is currently the number two ranked female billiards player in the world.

"It [the prohibitive back pain] hurts your confidence as well as your skill and focus," says Jeanette, who would like to practice more without pain and to regain the number one ranking. Though her present condition is detrimental to her ability to play pool, having surgery would fully prevent her from playing the game for an entire year and would permanently alter the range of motion she has in her back.

While Jeanette's scoliosis inhibits her development as a competitor, it is, in part, responsible for her ability to maintain a striking sense of humility despite the fame and accolade she has achieved in life.

"I'm just as human as everyone else," Jeanette says candidly. "I have a scar; I experience pain and depression. . . . [But] when these bad things happen, you have two choices—you can pity yourself, or you can overcome the problem. I've chosen the second." Her actions illustrate her choice, as she has never missed a tournament.

"You just work your way around these things to survive," Jeanette says of her scoliosis and her related back pain.

Not only has Jeanette decided to "work around" her scoliosis instead of letting it overcome her, but she has decided to utilize her fame and skill to benefit others with her condition. She has recently become a national spokesperson for the Scoliosis Association, Inc. Also, in January 1998 she founded the Jeanette Lee Foundation, which benefits two causes—scoliosis research and scholarship funds. Jeanette holds events to raise money for scoliosis research. She also raises money for scholarship funds and stresses the importance of education, responsibility, and forming healthy relationships to children.

"When I was a kid, I couldn't talk to anyone about my scoliosis. I didn't know of anyone else who had it or of any support organizations," Jeanette recalls. "I want people with scoliosis to know that they can talk to someone . . . [that] they're just as beautiful as everyone else, and that there are people out there who do understand what they're going through."

I am sure the same determination and optimism that Jeanette has displayed in coping with her scoliosis will serve her well in regaining her title as the number one female pool player in the world.

You can contact Jeanette through her personal website at www.jeanettelee.com. *The website includes information about Jeanette's career, the various charities that she benefits, the events (charity or competitive) in which she participates, the products she endorses, and her media schedule.*

MICHELLE MAUNEY

Beauty Queen

Michelle is a blonde bombshell whose extraordinary poise is augmented by an easygoing friendliness and whose impressive eloquence is glazed with a charming southern accent. Looking at this former Miss North Carolina USA, you can tell why she is known to be a serial winner of bathing suit competitions. What you would never guess by looking at Michelle, though, is that she was born with congenital heart disease and scoliosis.

Six months after Michelle was born, her parents took her to the hospital for a routine checkup. Doctors then detected four heart defects with which Michelle had been born. Preoccupied with Michelle's heart disease, doctors did not notice that she had also been born with scoliosis. Doctors at the hospital told Michelle's parents that their daughter—their only child—would need heart surgery as soon as possible. It was a matter of life and death, for the four heart defects little Michelle was

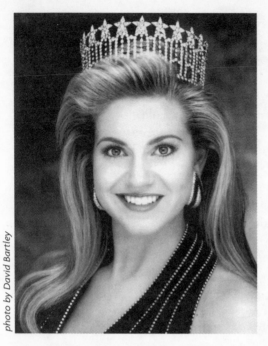

photo by David Bartley

plagued with, when left untreated, are known to kill during adolescence.

For the next few years, doctors monitored Michelle's health and awaited the day when Michelle would be strong enough to have heart surgery. At four, Michelle underwent a successful open heart surgery which, though it left her scarred, ensured that she would live a long, healthy life. Michelle quickly recovered from the heart surgery and soon became a very active child. She began kindergarten, made friends, and started to take dance classes. Michelle's strength of spirit made up for the relative weakness of her heart. And, although her heart was not as strong as everyone else's, it functioned correctly and served Michelle well.

When Michelle was six years old, she visited the hospital to have routine chest X rays. Doctors were pleased with the way Michelle's heart looked in the chest X rays. They were displeased, however, with the appearance of Michelle's spine in these X rays. It was at this doctor's visit that Michelle's doctors diagnosed her with scoliosis; they quickly realized that she had been born with scoliosis but that it had been too mild to detect at birth. Fearing that Michelle's scoliosis would progress, the doctors immediately put her into a back brace. For the next eight years, Michelle would wear her Boston low-profile back brace for twenty-three hours each day.

Though Michelle's parents knew the back brace she received at age six would remain with her for the rest of her childhood, they proffered no qualms about or objections to Michelle's wearing the brace. Her parents understood the medical implications of this early scoliosis and that if the scoliosis increased, it would eventually cause a rotation of Michelle's ribs. This rotation of the ribs would, in turn, compress and compromise Michelle's heart and lungs. While this is a slightly foreboding prospect for the typical scoliosis patient, it was utterly frightening for Michelle and her family. Michelle's heart was already weak; it could not have stood the pressure that a severe scoliosis curve would have created. With this in mind, her parents and her doctors felt confident that bracing was the correct mode of treatment.

Michelle wore her back brace faithfully. Though having to wear a brace throughout her childhood became a great annoyance and a burden to Michelle, she knew that the purpose of the brace was critical so she was persistent in wearing it. Unfortunately, when Michelle was fourteen, doctors determined that the brace would not be enough to effectively detain her scoliosis curve. Michelle had a rapidly progressing scoliosis curve that would not stop until surgery was performed. Michelle and her parents were disappointed that Michelle's hard work in brace wearing had not paid off, but they tried to view Michelle's imminent surgery in a positive light. They knew that if Michelle did not have the surgery, she would eventually run into severe pain, deformity, and more heart problems; therefore, they followed the doctors' recommendation and scheduled Michelle's surgery.

At fourteen, after eight years of wearing a back brace, Michelle underwent a spinal fusion with a Luque instrumentation system, which was new on the market at the time. During the surgery, Michelle's doctors corrected her almost sixty-degree curve to a dramatically lesser measurement of about thirty degrees. Prior to the surgery, Michelle remembers having been scared. Afterwards, she remembers having been so glad that she had gone through with the surgery and so relieved that she would never have to wear her brace again. Michelle did not have to wear any sort of body cast or brace post-operatively, and she returned home from the hospital in two weeks. Though she felt some discomfort in her spine after her surgery, Michelle was more bothered by the discomfort in the part of her hip where doctors had taken the bone graft for the fusion. But the pain subsided as time progressed. Michelle was not allowed any physical activity for nine months after the surgery, and only after an entire year did she feel fully recovered. Michelle felt compelled to keep her body hidden from the world. She felt very self-conscious about the scars on her chest (from the heart surgery) and her back (from the scoliosis surgery). She never wanted to go swimming because she was too embarrassed to put on a bathing suit.

Gradually, Michelle gained confidence. Her friends and family were very supportive of her throughout her surgery and recovery. They understood that Michelle was self-conscious about her scars and consciously fostered Michelle's self-confidence. Michelle resumed dancing lessons after her spinal fusion; she took up tap, a form of dancing that did not require that much back flexibility. As she developed skill in tap dancing, Michelle was able to slowly build her self-confidence.

While Michelle was busy dancing, all of her friends seemed to be busy participating in local beauty pageants. For a long time Michelle's friends tried to convince her to join, but Michelle was hesitant. Finally, though, she came to a conclusion concerning the possibility of her participating in pageants. Just as jumping into a cold pool is the only way to face the icy water, joining a pageant was, to Michelle, the only way she could force herself to face and combat her defeating self-consciousness—once and for all.

Michelle entered into her first pageant, The Miss Mount Holly Pageant, when she was eighteen years old. To Michelle's surprise, despite the visible scars on her chest and back, she ended up winning the swimsuit competition! Moreover, she was the first runner-up for the entire pageant. These accomplishments filled Michelle with the self-confidence she had lacked for so many years and signified that she had jumped over a major hurdle (her self-consciousness) in her personal development. In her next pageant, The Miss Castonia Pageant, Michelle won the swimsuit competition once again. And, this time, she became the winner of the entire pageant. For some time, Michelle continued to compete in local-level pageants. She came to enjoy the pageants that her friends had originally needed to *force* her to participate in, and she seemed to be emerging as a star in the pageant world. Soon Michelle surpassed local-level pageants and started competing on the state level. And, in 1995, she became Miss North Carolina USA.

In her role as Miss North Carolina USA, Michelle took on a multitude of responsibilities that consumed her life. She had to suspend everything she was involved in—including her attendance at Belmont Abbey College in North Carolina. Michelle describes her year-long reign as a "whirlwind year."

When Michelle's reign as Miss North Carolina USA was over, she completed her college education and returned to volunteering for the Scoliosis Association, Inc. Presently, she travels all over the country doing motivational speaking. Michelle's platforms include the topics of "overcoming adversities," and "setting goals and achieving them." If anyone is qualified to speak about these issues, it is Michelle. In the face of congenital heart disease and scoliosis, she became a beautiful, outgoing pageant winner. She responsibly addressed and accepted the adversity she was handed by fate, struggled with the self-doubt wrought by that adversity, and emerged as the winner of that struggle.

Scoliosis-related discrepancies in Michelle's hips and shoulder blades still exist because her curve was only corrected to thirty degrees and not to zero degrees. (In almost all scoliosis cases, people still have curvature in their spines after surgery. The curvature after surgery is just a lot less than it was before surgery, and the spine is prevented from curving any further.) She tries to cover the obvious asymmetries in her body with the clothes she chooses to wear. Though, to look at Michelle, one would never suspect any asymmetry. When she enters a room, her beauty and gentility command attention.

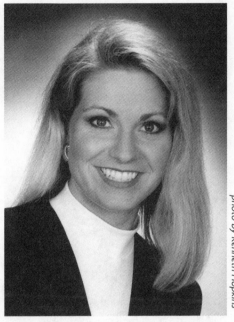

photo by Kenneth Hopkins

KELLY PATTEN

Rising Gymnastics Star

Kelly was only three years old when she began taking gymnastics. Almost immediately, she excelled in her "Tiny Tots" class and demonstrated a natural talent for the sport. Since then, Kelly has always been a step ahead of herself in gymnastics. Always moving up in the rankings, Kelly has never had trouble keeping up in practice sessions with much older girls. When she was five, Kelly was one of the few talented children in her "Gymbees" class to be moved into the group of six-year-olds. At six, Kelly began working out with the preteen group for four

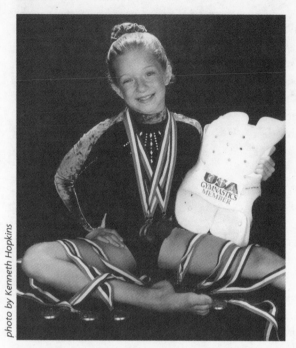

photo by Kenneth Hopkins

of the several hours she spent at the gym each week. At age seven, Kelly stepped up her pace once again and started to practice with the pre-teens for six of the many hours she spent at the gym each week.

One day in August 1996, Kelly's mother Robin was picking up eight-year-old Kelly after her gymnastics practice. When Robin walked into the gym, Kelly's gymnastics coach approached her and expressed a concern he had about Kelly. The coach pointed out to Robin some notable asymmetries in Kelly's body. He told her that Kelly had been favoring her right ankle in practice lately, and that he was able to see a hump in Kelly's back that was visible through her leotard. The coach was worried about Kelly and recommended that Robin take her to see a doctor. Luckily, Kelly was scheduled to have a pre-third grade checkup with her pediatrician in about a week.

The following week, Kelly and Robin found themselves in Kelly's pediatrician's office. Thinking that Kelly's preference for landing on her right ankle and the hump her coach had detected in her back were good points to address but not points of concern, Robin casually mentioned the gymnastics coach's findings to the pediatrician. Both Robin and Kelly were surprised when the pediatrician concluded from her visual examination of Kelly that Kelly was experiencing "the onset of early stages of scoliosis." The pediatrician immediately referred Kelly and her mother to a sports medicine orthopedic doctor at a nearby hospital and recommended that Kelly have X rays taken and a thorough examination.

A few days later, Robin took Kelly to see the recommended orthopedic surgeon. After performing a visual examination of Kelly, the orthopedic doctor agreed with the pediatrician in saying that Kelly was experiencing the onset of early stages of scoliosis. He told Robin that Kelly's scoliosis was not very significant in magnitude and that he wouldn't recommend any sort of treatment for it just yet. Still, the orthopedic doctor asked Robin and Kelly to remain at the hospital long enough to have X rays of Kelly's spine taken; he just wanted to be sure that his assessment of the situation was correct.

Kelly's X-rays illustrated that she had a fourteen-degree thoracic curve and a twenty-degree lumbar curve. The doctor was glad he had waited to see X rays before sending Kelly home, for the X rays showed what the simple, visual examination could not; Kelly's scoliosis was a lot more serious than the doctor had thought it was. Upon seeing these X rays, the orthopedic doctor explained to Kelly and her mother that this was a case of juvenile idiopathic scoliosis—meaning that it had no known cause (except, possibly, genetics). He told Kelly and Robin that Kelly did not need any treatment yet. He said that he would wait to document some progression of the curve before he put Kelly into a brace. In the meantime he warned them that, within six months to a year, Kelly would *probably* be wearing a back brace to treat her scoliosis.

In December 1996, four months after her original diagnosis, Kelly returned to the orthopedist have more X rays taken. These X rays illustrated that Kelly's thoracic curve was now fifteen degrees and that her lumbar curve was now twenty-three degrees. The doctor told Kelly and Robin that he still felt that bracing was not yet necessary. He asked Kelly and her mother to return to the hospital in four more months and forewarned them that at that time, bracing would be required.

Though a back brace sometime in the near future appeared inevitable, Kelly did not get upset or angry. She forgot about her scoliosis for the next four months and concentrated on her gymnastics. Kelly was so busy excelling at gymnastics—the single most important thing in her life—that she did not even realize that four months had gone by.

In April, Kelly and Robin found themselves, once again, in the office of their orthopedic doctor. From December 1996 to April 1997, Kelly had grown three quarters of an inch and had gained two pounds. Moreover, new X rays showed that her scoliosis had increased. Her thoracic curve had moved from fifteen degrees to twenty degrees and her lumbar curve had moved from twenty-three degrees to twenty-four degrees. To Kelly's and Robin's surprise, their doctor told them that bracing was *still* not necessary for Kelly. He told them to return for an examination, once more, in another four months. Kelly and Robin left the doctor's office feeling very excited that day. They had anticipated that the doctor would tell them that Kelly needed a brace at that appointment, but, fortunately, they had been wrong.

The bliss Kelly and her parents felt after having been told that Kelly did not yet need to be braced would not last for very long. By August 1997, Kelly had grown another inch and X rays showed that her scoliosis curves were now equal to one another, measuring twenty-four degrees each. At her August 1997 doctor's visit, nine-year-old Kelly was told that she needed to be braced, and Robin was given the name of an orthotist whom the doctor recommended. Though they had been discussing bracing for about a year, Kelly and her family realized now, once they actually had the brace in their hands, that talking about bracing is completely different than actually *having* a brace.

"I think we went home and were sort of shocked. We didn't know what to think until we actually went [to the orthotist's office] and saw the brace and the photographs of children wearing the brace and saw that you couldn't tell [that the children in the photographs were wearing back braces]. Kelly was extremely quiet on the ride home that day. There were no tears until Kelly came home with her brace. [Then] she was extremely weepy and unhappy to be wearing it because it was so uncomfortable."

Kelly's brace had been fitted so that her twenty-four-degree thoracic curve measured five degrees while she was in the brace and her twenty-four-degree lumbar curve measured ten degrees while she was in the brace. Kelly was bound to be uncomfortable in a brace that pushed her spine into such a straight position; after all, she was used to having her spine curved at this point. But the tightness of this brace would prove to be the most effective in halting the progression of Kelly's scoliosis curve; therefore, it would not be loosened at all.

To help Kelly get used to her back brace, her doctor invited her to a class, given at the hospital, on how to care for the brace. Half of the people in the class had just been fitted for their first back braces; half had just been fitted for their second back braces (these were kids who had already grown out of their first braces). Just seeing how many other children had to wear braces and how many children had already moved on to their second braces made Kelly feel better about wearing her own brace. During this class, Kelly and Robin learned many useful tricks for brace wearing, including how to line dry the t-shirts worn under the brace instead of putting them in the dryer so that they would not shrink and how to use Gold Bond Powder on the skin to prevent irritation from the brace. Kelly was also given a printed schedule for weaning herself into brace wearing over a two-week period. The schedule started with a few hours of brace wearing each day and gradually worked patients up to twenty-three hours of brace wearing each day. Robin thought that this schedule and this weaning process really helped Kelly to adjust to the brace and to ease herself into wearing it. After her day spent at the hospital, Kelly was much more comfortable with her brace and much more relaxed about having to wear it.

"Then one month [after Kelly had started wearing] the brace," Robin remembers, "Kelly became very uncomfortable and her left lateral rib was becoming very red and irritated and painful underneath. The rubbing alcohol and powder that we would put on it weren't working. I finally called [the orthotist's office] and said they needed to look at it. We went up and what they found was that [Kelly] had grown a little bit, and the padding wasn't pushing where it needed to be pushing; it needed to be readjusted. So they re-adjusted it, and that was very successful."

Once she had overcome all of her initial brace-related difficulties and had made all of the adjustments she needed to make in order to feel comfortable in her brace, Kelly had very little trouble with her brace. She began wearing it for her required twenty-three-hour-a-day regimen and made exceptions to her schedule only for gymnastics practice. Having a brace has in no way inhibited Kelly from pursuing gymnastics. She remains the energetic, committed, talented little girl she was prior to her getting the back brace.

Since she has been in her brace, Kelly has continued to meet success in the world of gymnastics. Her coach made the decision, with her parents, to move Kelly into level six gymnastics—a level very high for a gymnast so young. As a third grader, Kelly was practicing gymnastics for ten hours a week (when she was not wearing her brace) and competing in level six competitions. Since then, Kelly has gone to various state competitions and has won several gold and silver medals. Recently Kelly, now ten years old, qualified to compete in the state championships, where she won second place for her all-around performance, in addition to winning three bronze medals in other events.

Kelly never neglects to wear her brace; she wears it to school, to friends' houses, and everywhere else she goes. One of the elements in Kelly's life that has made brace wearing much easier for her to endure is her school environment. While Kelly was weaning herself into her new brace, she was also starting a new school. Concerned about the reaction of Kelly's schoolmates to her brace, Kelly's parents decided to speak to some of the school's faculty and administration about the issue. The school recommended a particular teacher for Kelly whose own daughter happened to have some medical problems. The teacher suggested that Kelly and her mother do a presentation about scoliosis for Kelly's class.

"It was like a little science lesson," Robin says. "Kelly drew the diagram on the board and we showed the kids how *her* spine looked [and then] how your spine *should* look. She lifted her shirt up and showed the class her brace. Children don't mean to be mean, but if they don't know what might be under her shirt, then they're left to talk and whisper and laugh. So rather than have Kelly feel like she was being whispered or talked about behind her back, we felt we'd answer everybody's questions all at once. We told the class [about the brace], and . . . the class asked if they could feel it. So Kelly walked around, and the class felt the brace and asked questions." After Kelly and Robin's presentation, the kids in Kelly's class were well-informed about scoliosis; they never whispered or talked about Kelly behind her back, and Kelly felt a lot more comfortable at her new school.

For a few months, Kelly juggled school, gymnastics, and brace-wearing without any problems. In December, though, approximately four months after receiving her brace, Kelly, as well as her family, began to tire of the brace, the scoliosis, and the mental and emotional toll the disorder was taking on their family.

"By December Kelly, her Dad, and I were coming to a little bit of a breaking point with trying to, I think, hit this problem head-on by ourselves as a family. We felt that we probably needed to reach for some sort of support," Robin says.

At the same time, Kelly's grandmother happened to see a television program featuring a member of a local scoliosis support organization. She contacted Kelly's parents and gave them the telephone number that had appeared on the television screen. Kelly and Robin decided to go to a meeting held by the organization, and since then they have been attending meetings every month. Knowing others who have scoliosis has helped Kelly's family to deal with her scoliosis and her brace.

Robin, Carl, and Kelly are all feeling more comfortable with Kelly's scoliosis, her brace, and the future possibility of surgery now that they have found a dependable source of support.

A Day in the Life of Kelly

- Sleep with the brace on.
- Take it off for breakfast.
- Put it back on at 8:00 A.M.
- Take the brace off for gym (though doctors say that she can partici- pate with it on, her gym teachers prefer that she takes it off for the safety of her and others); go to the school nurse for help taking the brace off and putting it back on.
- At 3:00 P.M., time for homework; take the brace off sometimes.
- At 5:00 P.M., go to the gym to practice gymnastics for three and a half hours—without the brace.
- At 8:45 P.M., eat dinner and then put the brace back on until morning.

At ten years of age, Kelly is a straight-A student and a very popular child. She never has problems with the children at school, and her friends are very supportive of her. They even like to help Kelly tighten her brace sometimes! Kelly recently received a Good Citizenship Award and Presidential Fitness Award. And, as always, Kelly excels at gym- nastics. This very determined ten-year-old plans to continue her devo- tion to wearing her back brace because she knows that it is the only thing warding off surgery for as long as possible. Though she feels uncomfortable in her brace sometimes, her love of gymnastics fully transcends any complaints she may have about her brace. Kelly's spir- ited outlook on life and devotion to her passion make it easy for her to treat her scoliosis actively and effectively.

CELEBRITIES WITH SCOLIOSIS

Yo-Yo Ma

For those of you who have not yet heard his name or his music, Yo-Yo Ma is a world-renowned cellist. Yo-Yo had scoliosis and was operated on several years ago by Dr. John Hall, who was a pioneer in the field of scoliosis and who now works at Boston Children's Hospital. A recent letter I received from the office of Yo-Yo Ma states that Yo-Yo "is one of Dr. Hall's very grateful patients . . . [and] feels it important that Dr. Hall be recognized for his work."[14] What Yo-Yo may not know is that he is an inspiation to all those who have scoliosis. He accepted his scoliosis, treated his curvature by means of undergoing surgery, and still found the strength to go on to become, perhaps, the best cellist in the world.

Isabella Rossellini

Isabella Rossellini, the daughter of actress Ingrid Bergman, has scoliosis. In her recent autobiography, *Some of Me*, she writes, "When I was eleven years old, I was diagnosed with scoliosis. I stood naked except for my underwear in a long queue of girls in the school gym. A doctor was to examine all of us. . . . [He said to me], 'Tell your parents . . . you have scoliosis, a deformity of the spine.'"

"To correct my scoliosis," Isabella continues, "I was attached to a special machine by the neck and the hips and pulled in opposite directions. Once the maximum correction was obtained, I was put into a cast. . . . After four months of this treatment, my S-shaped spine was corrected and fixed straight with an operation that consisted of a bone transplant taken from my leg. Thirteen of my vertebrae were fused together."[15]

Despite the trying experience she was forced to endure as a child, Isabella emerged to be a model, an actress, a mother, and an author. You have undoubtedly seen her face—often termed one of the most beautiful in the world—in advertisements for clothes and cosmetics and on television and movie screens. Though Isabella's scoliosis apparently had a huge impact on her childhood and her inner self, she did not *allow* it to have an impact on the course of her life or on her career. Despite having what she calls a "deformity" as a child, Isabella Rossellini grew up to be one of the most successful and well-known model-actresses in the world.

Interestingly, Isabella's teenage daughter, Elektra, has inherited her mother's scoliosis. Isabella regretfully mentions in her book that Elektra is now being treated for her scoliosis. And so continues the mystery of genetics.

Rene Russo

A magazine article about Rene Russo once stated, "In her childhood [Rene] had scoliosis and was so given to brooding she was often silent. But in the decades since she escaped from her back brace and her social awkwardness, she's become accessible, even a cutup."[16]

A successful actress on the Hollywood scene, the beautiful Rene Russo has starred in movies including *In the Line of Fire*, *Tin Cup*, and *Lethal Weapon IV*. Though she has admitted to interviewers that her scoliosis caused her much angst as a child, Rene has successfully escaped the emotional distress her deformity placed on her and has moved on to pursue her dreams and to lead a wonderfully successful life.

Wendy Whelan

Wendy Whelan is one of New York City Ballet's premier ballerinas. A popular principal dancer in one of the finest ballet companies in the world, Wendy embodies virtuosity, balance, and control in her lithe movements and demonstrates her innate love for dance in her ceaseless energy and magnetic stage presence. As a young ballet dancer, I often traveled to New York City to see her perform. It wasn't until my own scoliosis was diagnosed that I came to learn that my idol, Wendy Whelan, and I share the same diagnosis. Watching Wendy dance, one would never guess that she has scoliosis; but this thirty-one-year-old prima ballerina has been dealing with her spine disorder since she was just twelve years old. An article in an issue of *Dance* magazine included an account of Wendy's bout with scoliosis.

"There I was," she said, "all of twelve years old and being told that what lay ahead of me—instead of a summer of dance—was a choice of surgery for my spinal curvature or weeks of traction and a brace. I wanted to dance so badly, none of these things were going to stop me. So I chose the traction and the brace."[17]

Wendy endured years of traction and time spent in a Milwaukee brace so she could avoid surgery and pursue her dream of dancing. She even attended ballet class during the time when she was in a body cast!

"I was the funniest looking thing in school," Wendy says of herself wearing a brace, "but I didn't care because I had a definite goal to reach."[18]

Once Wendy had reached skeletal maturity, she no longer had to worry about treating her scoliosis. She had been accepted into the New

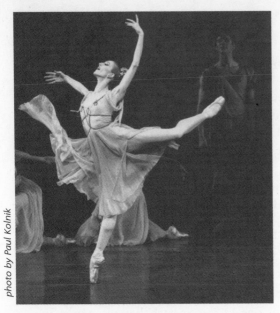

photo by Paul Kolnik

York City Ballet company and was more focused on her dancing career than on her spine. However, Wendy's struggle with scoliosis was not completely over.

During the course of our interview, Wendy revealed to me that she has experienced notable back pain throughout her dancing career and has had to work at keeping her body correctly placed and aligned. Luckily, New York City Ballet's physical therapists have developed a technique known as "body mirroring" to treat their dancers who have any degree of scoliosis. This treatment has apparently worked well to keep Wendy balanced and flexible and to keep her curvature in check. So, as Wendy Whelan continues to amaze audiences with her incredible skill and artistry, her scoliosis lies quietly beneath the surface. She has never allowed her scoliosis to inhibit her pursuit of her passion, and it does not look like it ever will. A lovely, serene lady on stage as well as off, Wendy Whelan inspires more awe in me than than ever before.

Chapter 4

Surgery: When It Comes to This

I n considering surgery as a treatment option for your scoliosis, you must first ask yourself, "When does surgery become necessary?" In trying to find the answer to this question, you will inevitably come across other questions, such as: "Who has the qualifications and knowledge to tell me that surgery is necessary?" "What degree of curvature necessitates surgery?" "Can a person be too young or too old to have surgery?" "What are the implications of surgery?" and "Is there any suitable alternative to having surgery?"

The single most important thing to know when you are considering surgery is that the majority of scoliosis surgeries are elective. This means that, in most cases, the patient has the opportunity to decide whether or not to have surgery and when to have surgery. Rarely is a scoliosis-related spinal fusion a "life-or-death" matter or even a matter of urgency, especially if it is an idiopathic curve in an adolescent or adult patient. Growing children (infants and juveniles) with severe curves may also be candidates for early surgical intervention. It is likely that you will have several months, several years, or even a lifetime to mull over the decision of whether or not to have surgery for your scoliosis. Remember, though, that the factors you must consider regarding surgery (*i.e.*, degree of curvature, age, flexibility of spine, and overall health; see chapter 5) will change as the months and years pass.

Urgent surgery is usually called for when a spinal rotation is so severe that it can seriously decrease lung capacity or compromise another organ, such as your heart; when your scoliosis-related pain is so acute that it is prohibitive to everyday living; or when you are deformed to a degree that makes it difficult for you to walk or to partake in other simple aspects of everyday living.

In the majority of cases, though, surgery is elective. In determining whether this elective surgery is appropriate for you, you must consider factors such as the flexibility of your spine, your degree of curvature, and your skeletal maturity and/or age. In addition to these factors, other important factors include the amount of pain you feel, your pulmonary function, your deformity or appearance, and your overall health.

As a general rule, doctors do not like to perform surgery on patients who are very young (infant to age ten) or those who are in their later adulthoods (age sixty-five and older). If you are very young and have not yet finished growing, a fusion of your spine will "weld" together your vertebrae so that it will no longer grow in length with the rest of your body. If you are an older patient, your spine is less flexible and your body less resilient; these factors threaten to make surgery more complicated and recovery more prolonged and painful. On the other hand, maybe you are a thirteen-year-old who has stopped growing; perhaps you are a sixty-five-year-old whose body and bones resemble those of a fifty-five-year-old. Cases such as these exhibit exceptions to the rule—and there are, of course, exceptions to every rule.

Lifestyle, age, skeletal maturity, curve magnitude, flexibility of spine, degree of pain, severity of deformity, and overall health are factors that vary indefinitely. Each scoliosis case is unique. You must be responsible for weighing all of the factors that are important to you and decide if surgery is the answer. Your doctor is likely to have a great influence in your decision-making, but remember: a single doctor's opinion, while invaluable, is just one part of the research you need to determine whether or not you should have surgery. In my opinion, it is not just important, but *necessary* to seek two, three, or even four doctors' opinions before deciding which treatment path to take. This way, you will get a feel for the options that are open to you.

GETTING SECOND AND THIRD OPINIONS

Most of the time, a doctor is the one who will inform you that "surgery is necessary." Even if the doctor who tells you this has been your only doctor for several years, you should seek other doctors' opinions before heading into the operating room. Remember that doctors' opinions may vary. One doctor may think that you need surgery right away, while another may think that you can wait for another few months or even years. One doctor may want to fuse several levels of your spine while another may decide only to fuse fewer levels of your vertebrae, thereby sparing valuable motion levels. One doctor may want to use one continuous rod for the length of your entire fusion, while another may want to use a series of rods with multiple anchors (segmental). One doctor may want to put you into a brace after surgery, while another may not.

Seeking more than one opinion not only introduces you to the various possibilities available to you, but it gives you knowledge about your curve, about scoliosis, and about different surgical techniques. It ensures that you will not blindly fall into having surgery; on the other hand, it may enable you to find a doctor who will perform surgery when others have refused. It also allows *you* to be in charge of making the decisions about the possibility of having surgery. After you have sought several opinions, you are in a position to compare the opinions, to weigh the validity of each, and to choose which you think is right for you.

BROOKE

My thoracic curve measured forty degrees and my lumbar forty-two when I turned sixteen and reached skeletal maturity in the fall of 1996. The only thing I could do at this point, doctors told me, was to wait. After a year, they would take new X rays of my spine and would determine whether any progression had occurred.

Throughout the following year, I focused on school, ballet, and other things. Since I was no longer wearing a brace, I found it easy to let the issue of my scoliosis slip to the back of my mind. At times, I would completely forget about my scoliosis, thinking that it was a thing of the past. But the periodic muscle spasms I had in my back, the alterations I had to have made in my clothes, and the appearance of my back—including asymmetric muscles, a protruding scapula, and an obviously curved spine—were always present to remind me of my scoliosis. And although I knew well that surgery was a very real possibility for me, I somehow entertained the idea that I was done treating my scoliosis and that I would never require surgery. I saw my mildly disfigured body and felt the pain in my back muscles, but never *truly* acknowledged that my curvature might be worsening; I attributed these symptoms to the curvature I already knew I had.

In preparing to write this book, I decided that I should have a first-hand look at scoliosis from a medical point of view. During the summer of 1997, I was doing research and gaining experience by way of an externship I did with a spine surgeon at a local hospital. I followed this surgeon around the hospital, visiting scoliosis clinics with him and observing scoliosis surgeries. Seeing scoliosis patients and their X rays every day, I could not help but wonder about the present condition of my own spine. By August of that summer, I was growing impatient. I needed to know whether my scoliosis had progressed.

Almost a year had passed since I had obtained my last set of X rays. The doctor posted my new X rays on the viewing box immediately and began discussing them.

My thoracic curve had progressed to forty-nine degrees, and my lumbar curve had progressed to fifty-one degrees. Despite the fact that I had finished growing for quite a while, my scoliosis was worsening. Of course I knew that this meant that my scoliosis would worsen indefinitely, yet slowly, until I had surgery. Though I had known that this was a viable possibility, I had never really confronted the idea of it. Now, though, my need to have surgery was a reality that I would have to face.

When the doctor said the words, "You definitely need to have surgery," I was neither shocked nor surprised, but I certainly experienced an unexpected moment of disappointment and realization. I sat quietly on the examining table, feeling sad about the future of my dancing and annoyed by the fact that I would have to disrupt my life to have and recover from this surgery. I thought about the people I knew who had undergone surgery and about how quickly they had recovered and how well they had faired. I told myself that I knew so much about surgery now that there was nothing for me to fear. And I convinced myself that I had no right to be upset by the fact that I needed surgery; though surgery had just been a possibility and not a reality beforehand, I had had years to get used to the *idea*. So I begrudgingly accepted my fate and listened to what the doctor had to say.

Opinion #1: Pointing to the X ray on the viewing box, the doctor told me that if *he* were to do the surgery, he would fuse both the thoracic and lumbar curves (almost the entire length of my spine) posteriorly, except a few lower lumbar levels.

"Yup," he said, "we can just go in there and zip you all the way up— we can make the whole thing straight! You're so flexible that your curves will straighten really well. It will be beautiful; just one long, thin scar down your whole back."

At this, my mother and I tried to convince the doctor that I had *no* interest in having such a long, solid fusion. While the doctor seemed to be marveling at the thought of doing a full-length fusion and creating a long, straight, fused spine, I was cringing at the idea of the loss of motion this approach to surgery would occasion.

"I don't mind having the surgery," I said to the doctor. "I won't mind the recovery, and I don't care about scars or anything like that. The only thing I ask is that every measure is taken to maintain as much of my range of motion as possible. The only thing I care about with respect to my surgery is my future ability to dance."

Still, though, the doctor maintained that the approach he had suggested was the only surgical approach he found appropriate or would consider in my case. My mother and I graciously thanked him for his opinion and told him that we would have to get a second opinion before making a decision. He encouraged us to get a second opinion, arranging for us to take the new X rays from his office to the office of another doctor. My mother and I thanked this doctor for his giving us the X rays and for his being so understanding. We left the hospital, hoping to find a doctor who would propose a different approach to my imminent surgery.

Opinion #2: Within a week following my first encounter with the prospect of surgery, I saw a second doctor. Though this doctor agreed with the first doctor's conclusion that I needed surgery, he was much more understanding of my lifestyle and my love for dance. He looked carefully at my X rays and listened closely when I told him that my primary concern about having surgery was losing the range of motion in my back. Accordingly, this doctor proposed an approach to surgery that would correct my scoliosis without compromising my range of motion. He said that if *he* were to do the surgery, he would fuse my spine from the T12 vertebra to the L2 vertebra; this meant he would only be fusing one of my two curves. This doctor explained that if one curve was fused, the other *should* naturally correct itself so that it would balance the surgically straightened curve. In addition, this doctor proposed doing an anterior approach to my surgery. He said that, by doing my surgery from the front of my spine rather than from the back, he would be able to preserve much of the flexibility in my spine.

After thoroughly discussing this approach to surgery and its implications with the second doctor, my parents and I decided that this surgery was an ideal option for me. This appointment took place in August 1997. Having faith in this doctor to perform a surgical process that would allow me to dance afterwards, my parents and I scheduled my surgery for the following June.

Opinion #3: In December 1997, I coordinated a special benefit performance of the *Nutcracker* by the New England Ballet Company. The ballet, in which I danced the lead role, was followed by a gala reception. A scoliosis surgeon I had heard about but had never met was in attendance at the performance and gala that night. Many people had previously told me that this doctor was a world-renowned leader in his field; many had told me that I should seek his opinion about my condition. And I had considered visiting this doctor, but I had not yet had the time or the need to do so.

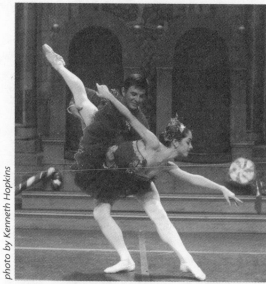

photo by Kenneth Hopkins

Brooke Lyons and Bill Pizzuto perform the Grand Pas de Deux in the Nutcracker.

The gala reception that evening was my first opportunity to meet this doctor, and I was shocked to hear him say, upon meeting me, "I don't think you have to have surgery yet." This renowned surgeon had seen me dance and had seen the appearance of my back in the low-backed dress I was wearing at the gala.

"You should come to my office to see me," he said. Pleasantly surprised but careful not to get my hopes up, I promised I would pay him a visit before having surgery in June.

That February, my mother and I traveled to see this doctor. We carried with us the same X rays I had obtained in August from the first doctor, who had recommended surgery. After examining these X rays, this third doctor remeasured them and determined that my curves did *not* measure forty-nine and fifty-one degrees, as the first doctor had told me. This doctor was adamant in concluding that my thoracic curve actually measured forty-three degrees and my lumbar curve forty-seven degrees! He explained that the other doctor (the first one) must have erred in drawing the Cobb angles on my X rays.

Even though he had discovered that my curves were slightly less severe than I had been told, he confirmed that surgery was still necessary. Contrary to what the other doctors had said, though, this doctor did not feel that surgery was necessary *immediately*. He knew about my love of dancing—after all, he had seen me perform—and was very concerned about how surgery would affect my back flexibility and my ability to dance. Furthermore, he told me that my spine was so flexible that he could attain the same degree of correction if he performed surgery now, or if he performed it a couple of years from now. For these reasons, he suggested I wait until my scoliosis became more severe and surgery was unequivocally necessary. We agreed to keep a close eye on my spinal deformity with periodic (yearly) X rays to be sure my scoliosis wouldn't increase to degrees of unnecessary severity.

What I really appreciated was that this doctor was not looking at me as a statistic or even as a patient; he was looking at me as a person. In making his decision, he not only took into account my curve magnitude, spine flexibility, and skeletal maturity; he also took into account my interests and my lifestyle. Again, I can't emphasize enough the importance of selecting a surgeon who considers the total person.

He also suggested a surgical approach different than had been previously suggested. He rejected the approach of the first doctor, saying that fusing my entire spine would be gratuitous. He rejected the approach of the second doctor, saying that an anterior approach would not give me the solidity of fusion I needed and that fusing so few vertebrae and *expecting* my second curve to straighten on its own would risk a second surgery. In his opinion, the appropriate surgical approach to my curve at this point in time would be to fuse my spine posteriorly from T8 to L2—subject to change with curve pattern and new developments in surgical techniques as my surgery becomes imminent.

Having spent several hours consulting this third surgeon on the future treatment of my scoliosis, I decided to cancel the scheduled June 1998 surgery date.[18]

As you can see from my experience, doctors' opinions of and approaches to situations *will* vary. If I had agreed with the first doctor who recommended surgery, I would now have most of my spine fused and would be unable to bend very much or to dance. Because I sought other opinions and thoroughly researched the options open to me, though, I have not yet had surgery and am still dancing today. My scoliosis is increasing slowly, but my doctor feels that if I wait a few more years to have surgery, with periodic followup, I will still attain the same amount of correction and will have just as uncomplicated a surgery and recovery process as I would have if I had surgery today.

Since surgery is a fairly imminent prospect for me, I am thankful to have this time to live and dance freely. While I know that my life will be changed and my ability to dance altered forever, I am very thankful just to *have* a few more years to dance.

What to Do if Opinions Vary

When you seek several doctors' opinions about whether or not surgery is the right treatment for you or about which surgical technique would suit your body and your curve the best, you will inevitably come across differences—even direct contradictions—in the various opinions you receive. If you have received a variety of doctors' opinions and are confused as to which doctor you should believe, you can do one of three things.

1. Continue to see doctors until one opinion emerges as the prevalent opinion. In general, when a couple of different doctors suggest a particular treatment or surgical technique for you, that treatment or surgical technique is probably the right one.
2. Research scoliosis and surgical techniques on your own. Read about surgery, ask doctors questions about surgery, present doctors with suggestions that other doctors have given you, and utilize every available outlet of information concerning scoliosis surgery. Then make the right decision (pertaining to surgery) for yourself based on what you know and what the doctor(s) whom you trust the most has/have told you.

3. Take the "easy way out" *(not recommended)*[20] and return to the doctor whose opinion you liked best.

Over time, as you gather information, hear various opinions, and become more informed about scoliosis and scoliosis surgery, you will feel better equipped to make a decision. Never rush into having surgery performed by a doctor whose suggested surgical approach you do not like. On the other hand, do not avoid having surgery because you have convinced yourself that you have not or will never find an opinion that suits you. Try to be honest with yourself, open to various suggestions, aware of your condition, and as rational as you can be, considering that discussing surgery is a process tinted by various shades of emotion. And, most important, remember that the confusion you feel after having heard several conflicting opinions *will* eventually subside. Ultimately, you will know which approach to surgery is right for you, and it is not until then that you should head into the operating room.

RISKS AND BENEFITS OF SURGERY

Surgery carries with it certain risks that should be anticipated and, if possible, avoided. These risks include the following:

◆ Pseudarthrosis, or failure of the fusion to take place, in which case your newly straightened spine might be fragile or likely to curve if there are no implants in your spine, or cause implants to break if you have them. (This is uncommon in adolescent patients and is more likely to occur in older patients, smokers, and patients undergoing revision surgery.)

◆ An injury to your neurological structures (*i.e.*, paralysis from an injury to the spinal cord). Studies show that this sort of risk materializes in less than one in one thousand surgeries performed.

◆ A post-operative infection of your wound/incision.

◆ Failure of the instrumentation to hold, in which case you would either leave broken/loosened rods in your back or have surgery to remove them. This is usually the result of a nonunion, decreased spine strength, or improperly placed implants.

◆ Decompensation[21] following surgery. This is more likely to occur in instances where a selective thoracic fusion is performed. In other words, if you have a thoracic curve and a lumbar curve, and your doctor just fuses your thoracic curve in hopes that your lumbar curve will compensate by straightening on its own, you risk having your lumbar curve remain curved and your body unbalanced. Such decompensation has been reported in up to twenty percent of patients treated with selective thoracic fusion techniques. Post-operative bracing often corrects these decompensation problems, and a very small minority of patients require an extension of the fusion into the lumbar spine (more surgery).

◆ For adolescents, a fusion of certain vertebrae—especially if a significant number of lumbar vertebrae are involved—is a transfer of stress to the unfused vertebrae. This, coupled with the age-related changes of degeneration, can lead to instability and pain. (The sooner your vertebrae are fused, the sooner the rest of your spine stops moving as much, and the sooner you begin your journey toward eventual arthritic changes in your unfused spine segments.)

While there is no surefire way to avoid falling victim to the risks that accompany surgery, there are many measures you can take in an attempt to protect yourself from such risks. Before having surgery, you should check with your doctor to make sure that you will have a neurological monitor and a specialist standing by this monitor in the operating room throughout your surgical process. The most commonly used neurological monitor during scoliosis surgery is the SSEP (Somato Sensory Evoked Potential). The SSEP is supplemented to the wake up test to evaluate motor function. More recently, the technique of monitoring the anterior (motor) pathway of the spinal column is under development and testing in some centers. This way, the person working the monitor will be able to alert your doctor if any changes from the baseline occur during surgery.

After surgery, make an effort to keep your incision or wound clean and protected to reduce your risk of contracting an infection. Cleansing solutions such as alcohol should be applied until the incision is healed.

THE PROS AND CONS OF SURGERY

Pros

- You will have a straighter spine.
- Once a solid fusion is achieved, your scoliosis will never progress again, and you will no longer have to worry about treating it.
- You decrease the risk of jeopardizing the health of your heart, lungs, and even your general health. This applies mostly to thoracic curves.
- Your appearance will be improved. Surgery will either lessen or completely rid you of embarrassing "humps," unevenness in your hips, differences in your shoulder heights, protrusion of one scapula, creases in your waist, and so on.
- If you have surgery sooner than later (at a younger age, or when your curve is not yet extremely severe), the entire procedure will be easier and recovery time reduced. The spine is more flexible and easier to straighten, and you will have increased resilience.
- You may get rid of scoliosis-related pain.
- You will feel more balanced and centered, and improve your sense of self.

Cons

- The "arthritis timeclock" starts when your spine is fused. In other words, the day of your surgery marks the beginning of a gradual decline in flexibility and the gradual degeneration of unfused motion segments. The more levels that are fused, the fewer lumbar levels remain, and the faster the decline.
- You cannot return to your "normal" activity level until one year after your surgery.
- You may never be able to play contact sports (or things that might harm your instrumentation or fusion) after your surgery.
- You might have surgery and then, a few years later, find out about a wonderful, new, easy technique/instrumentation system from which you could have benefited had you waited.
- The pain felt after surgery, the difficult recovery period, and the time spent waiting to feel "normal" again are all unpleasant.
- As is the case with any surgery, you risk running into complications or problems both during and after the surgery.

Do not pick up heavy objects or rush into certain physical activities after surgery unless your doctor tells you it is safe to do so. If you really listen to your doctor's advice and remain mindful of your spine, your new instrumentation, and your new fusion, you will decrease your risk for failure of fusion or failure of instrumentation to occur.

There are many benefits to having surgery. In many cases, the matter that drives people to have surgery is repaired by the surgery. For instance, if chronic back pain drives you to have surgery for your scoliosis, the surgery will probably rid you of the pain. If your deformity drives you to have surgery, the surgery will probably lessen the deformity and improve your cosmetic appearance. And, in all cases, surgery will dramatically lessen the degree of curvature in your spine and will prevent you from worrying about any future progression of your scoliosis or any future scoliosis-related health risks.

Cosmetic improvement is a major benefit of scoliosis surgery. For most adolescents, surgery is recommended to stop and to correct the progression of deformity and the progression of curve magnitude. Based on the natural history of these curves, deformities exceeding fifty degrees in a growing adolescent have been shown to continue to progress during adulthood; therefore, surgery is advised to partially correct the deformity and prevent progression into adult life. The risk of untreated scoliosis in an adult includes pain from degenerative changes within the spinal joints, and for severe thoracic deformities, cardipulmonary compromise, strain on the heart, and functional disability. Having surgery will reduce, if not annihilate, these risks.

HOW TO FIND THE RIGHT SURGEON

Finding the right surgeon to perform your surgery is of crucial importance. You want a surgeon who has skill, experience, and credentials. The surgeon you choose should suggest a surgical approach that suits you; operate in a clean, efficient, well-respected hospital; advocate a post-surgery casting/bracing arrangement (*i.e.*, no post-surgical bracing) that suits you; cares about you, your interests, and your lifestyle as well as about your scoliosis; and have the right bedside manner. As a general rule, make sure that everything about your surgeon, the way he or she conducts himself, and the way he or she operates feels right to

---

QUESTIONS YOU SHOULD ASK ANY DOCTOR YOU SEE FOR YOUR SCOLIOSIS

- What treatment do you propose?
- (If the doctor recommends surgery) What surgical approach would you suggest?
- How many levels (which vertabrae) would you fuse?
- What rod/instrumentation system do normally you use?
- How long (how many hours) would the type of surgery you are suggesting take to complete?
- How many scoliosis surgeries do you do each month?
- Would other doctors and/or residents be assisting you during the surgery?

---

you. You need to trust your doctor and trust that all of the factors that are important to you are taken into consideration. In addition to the obvious medical factors, your doctor should care about your psychological well-being, your normal activity level, your schedule, your physical interests, and any other concerns you express.

A scoliosis surgeon is an orthopedic surgeon who specializes in scoliosis and other spine-related disorders. He or she should be board-certified or board-eligible in orthopedic surgery by the American Academy of Orthopedic Surgeons. Scoliosis surgery is a sub-specialty of orthopedic surgery and therefore requires special training just in the area of scoliosis. Your doctor should have completed a fellowship training in scoliosis. As there is no board certification for scoliosis per se, the Scoliosis Research Society acts more or less as a certifying board. Look for a doctor who is a member of the SRS. You can find a doctor in your area who is a member of this prestigious society by simply calling the society (see Resource Directory). You may also contact the American Academy of Orthopedic Surgeons website (www.aaos.com) for hospitals that have scoliosis fellowships. There are scoliosis specialists all over the country; oftentimes, however, they are concentrated in the more renowned spine centers such as San Francisco, St. Louis, the Hospital for Special Surgery in New York, and Minnesota, to mention a few.

Other aspects of a doctor you may want to investigate include whether your doctor will be assisted by residents and other doctors during the surgery. In teaching hospitals (which many good hospitals are), this is the case. Do not worry too much about this, because in most cases doctors just allow the residents to help with minor surgical roles—not to do the actual operation. But, just to be on the safe side, make clear to your doctor that you want *him/her* to be the one performing the actual surgery. Also, aside from the nature of the surgery, the amount of experience a doctor has in that particular procedure is the element that determines how long the surgery will take to complete. The longer you are lying on the operating table, the longer your body is "asleep" and the more difficult it is to "wake up" your body to begin your recovery. Ask your doctor about how many scoliosis surgeries he or she performs each month to give you an idea of his or her experience. Also, be sure to ask the expected length of time for your surgery. And, of course, one of the most important things to do is ask for patient recommendations about your doctor.

Traveling a Long Distance for Surgery

Traveling a long distance to have surgery can be somewhat of a hassle, but it is certainly possible. Janice (see page 161) traveled several times from Florida to Minnesota to have surgery. She always traveled by plane and not by car, but traveling *immediately* after surgery was never an issue for her because she and her husband rented an apartment in Minnesota. This way, Janice had a place to stay for a few months after surgery and was able to fly back to Florida once she was feeling up to it.

Many people, though, need to travel long distances home immediately after their surgeries. Airplanes may not be the best alternative for these people, for airplanes are very public, cramped, and often uncomfortable. A better choice for the patient may be to ride home in a car or other vehicle. In a car or van, patients can lie down for the ride, stop the vehicle whenever necessary (*i.e.*, to use a bathroom), and avoid being disturbed by the presence (including sights, sounds, and smells) of unfamiliar people.

ERIKA

Erika's family, though inexperienced when it came to transporting a post-surgical scoliosis patient, did an excellent job of transporting Erika from Maryland to Connecticut just days after her surgery.

After fifteen-year-old Erika had endured a joint anterior/posterior spinal fusion and a difficult recovery period, she was ready to go home. The only question was, how was Erika going to get home? Her insurance did not cover transportation, so she was unable to ride home in an airplane. Furthermore, an airplane would probably not have been able to accommodate Erika very well. Deciding that Erika was unable to return home in a normal car, Erika's mother, Denise, called two of her uncles and asked for help. The next day, these two elderly uncles drove to Maryland in a big recreational vehicle with a makeshift bed inside. The bed was covered with a soft, egg-crate mattress to help make Erika as comfortable as possible.

Erika was given pain medication and Dramamine to prevent motion sickness during the ride; they situated her in the makeshift bed, provided as much comfort as possible, and then departed for Connecticut. Denise rode in the vehicle; Erika's grandmother followed close behind in a car.

For the first four hours of the ride, Erika slept. During that time, Denise lay beside Erika and made a bedbar (siderail) out of her own body to prevent Erika from rolling around in the event of a bump. After four hours, the uncles stopped the recreational vehicle, and Denise took Erika to a restroom. Then Erika took another pill for her pain and went back to sleep for the remainder of the ride. At 2:00 A.M., Erika woke up at home. The ride had gone smoothly, and Erika had returned to Connecticut unruffled and happy to be home.

CAN PATIENTS WHO ARE STILL GROWING HAVE SURGERY?

Doctors do not recommend spine fusions for patients who have not finished growing. When you have a spinal fusion, your spine will be fused and prevented from growing further. While the posterior portion of your spine will be fused and motionless (if you have a posterior fusion), the anterior part of your spine, as well as the rest of your body, will continue to grow. A situation such as this can put you at risk for what is called the "crankshift phenomenon." This occurs when the anterior portion of your spine grows and lengthens while the posterior portion remains stagnant; this can result in deformity, imbalance, and difficulties with your spine.

This does not, however, mean that you cannot have surgery if you are still growing and need immediate surgery. A certain type of instrumentation, called subcutaneous instrumentation, is used for young children whose curves are severe enough to warrant surgery. Subcutaneous instrumentation is an expandable implant designed to accommodate growth. This type of implant is welded onto the areas where your curvature begins and ends. The subcutaneous rods—just like any other rods—extend the length of the area in-between the beginning and end of your curvature. Unlike other surgeries, though, surgeries done with subcutaneous rods do not include a fusion of the entire curve. While the rods are present to hold your spine, they are only reinforced by a bone-graft fusion at the ends of the curve. This way, your scoliosis can be partially corrected, and a major segment of your spine can still have the opportunity to grow. As you grow, you will undergo periodic surgeries (every six months or so) during which your implants will be lengthened to accommodate your growing spine. Ultimately, once you have stopped growing, it will be necessary to undergo a surgery during which bone graft will be used to fuse the remainder of the curve in a straight position and to supplement your instrumentation. This final step—the fusion—ensures that your scoliosis will not be able to progress in the future.

PEOPLE WHO HAVE EXPERIENCED THE WAY SURGERY USED TO BE

MARIANNE
"We may bend, but never break."

A dressmaker who was fitting Marianne's skirt first noticed the deformity. One of Marianne's hips seemed to be higher than the other, and the dressmaker found it unusually difficult to make the hemline of Marianne's skirt hang evenly. The dressmaker suggested to Marianne's mother that she take her daughter to a doctor. Marianne's mother took Marianne to an orthopedic doctor to find out what was the matter with her daughter's hips. It was at this doctor's visit that Marianne discovered she had scoliosis. Then, at the age of twelve, Marianne did not have a severe enough curvature to warrant any sort of immediate treatment. Her doctor recommended that she return to him to have X rays taken every six months. The doctor hoped that such frequent X rays would accurately document any progression of Marianne's scoliosis curvature.

Marianne buried her feelings about her scoliosis, for she was concerned about her parents' worries over her sister, who had Down's Syndrome. Once Marianne's doctor had seen that her scoliosis was progressing, he put her into a body cast in order to stabilize her curve. The weekend she was put into her body cast was a particularly snowy winter weekend, and everyone was outside sledding. On Monday, when Marianne appeared at school with a body cast on, someone started a rumor that she had been in a sledding accident over the weekend; Marianne did not deny it.

"I never said anything to let them [the kids at school] know that the rumor wasn't true," Marianne remembers. "I may have even said that it *was* true." Marianne liked the rumor better than she did the truth; in her opinion, it helped ease the trauma of having to wear a body cast as a seventh grader in 1960. Marianne continued to wear her body cast for a full six months before her doctor decided to order her a Milwaukee back brace instead. While she was in the body brace, Marianne tried to continue life as usual.

"I continued to play sports, and it was very uncomfortable because it [the body cast] would stick to my body, and it would hurt," Marianne says. "And it was unbelievable to try to get clothes that would fit over it."

When Marianne finally had her body cast removed, it was replaced with a metal back brace. Marianne only wore her Milwaukee brace for one year before her doctor recommended surgery. Despite Marianne's use of a body cast as well as a back brace, her curve was progressing. Therefore, when she was thirteen, her orthopedic doctor in Virginia recommended a scoliosis surgery that was being done in Delaware at the time. Marianne's parents wisely sought a second opinion.

The second doctor explained that Marianne was nearing the end of her growth cycle and that there was a good chance that her scoliosis would soon stabilize. Marianne's parents preferred this approach to their daughter's scoliosis and followed the second doctor's advice without seeking a third opinion to verify that the second opinion had been the right one. Marianne feels that her parents opted to forego the surgery because it would have required travel to either Texas or Delaware (for the surgery was not done in Virginia at that time) and a six-month hospital stay. Marianne's family could not finance a temporary four-person migration to either Texas or Delaware, and they felt that by sending just Marianne, or Marianne and one parent so far away, it would be harmful to the family unit. Marianne did not have surgery for her scoliosis; she stayed in Virginia and moved on to high school, determined not to let her scoliosis impinge on her life.

"I had a wonderful high school life," she says. Of all Marianne's high school experiences, one of the most memorable was being a majorette in the high school marching band.

"We had these tight, gold lamé uniforms, and it bothered me to see that my shoulders were uneven," she says. "So my mother took me to an orthopedic appliance place, and the people there made me a little padded piece for my lower shoulder. But that didn't really work out very well, so I didn't use it."

From that point on, instead of seeking cosmetic help, Marianne learned to cope with her deformity on her own. She pursued sewing as a hobby in high school and was, therefore, able to make clothes that looked stylish and camouflaged her deformity. After high school, Marianne moved on to college.

"I had a wonderful college life," she remembers. "I was very active and involved and so forth. I met my husband the second day of my freshman year, and though we didn't marry until we had graduated, it made for very idyllic times." Throughout her college life, as in her high school life, Marianne did not do anything to treat her scoliosis. She always noticed the hump in her back and the unevenness in her shoulders and hips, but she hadn't noticed that these deformities had worsened since she had reached skeletal maturity. Marianne's failure to notice the progression of her scoliosis was likely a result of her doctor's telling her—years ago—that her scoliosis would "stabilize" once she had stopped growing.

After college, Marianne and her husband moved to Florida, allowing her husband to pursue his career as an aerospace engineer. In Florida, Marianne was very active and experienced no back pain whatsoever. She soon became an assistant principal at a Florida middle school and was busy at work most of the time. Marianne attributes her complete lack of pain or physical inhibition to her curve's being an "S" curve; in other words, she had a thoracic curve and a lumbar curve (to the opposite direction) and was, therefore, "pretty well-balanced."

Throughout her twenties, Marianne never saw a doctor until she contracted pneumonia at the age of twenty-eight. The pneumonia affected the lower lobe of one of Marianne's lungs that was "pinched by [her] scoliosis." (The rotation of her spine created a corresponding rotation of her rib cage, which cramped her lungs.) The doctor who treated Marianne for her pneumonia directed her to have a lung function test, and when the test showed that Marianne's scoliosis was taking a toll on her pulmonary function, she knew that she would eventually have to do something about it. Doctors assured her that it would be all right to have children and *then* to address the issue of her scoliosis, but this brief encounter with the prospect of surgery brought Marianne closer to her scoliosis.

"It [scoliosis and the prospect of surgery] was definitely something staring me in the face now," she says.

In her thirties, Marianne experienced three natural childbirths. Through her pregnancies, she regretted having had X rays every six months during her early teenage years. Marianne knew now the dangers of frequent exposure to radiation that neither she nor her doctor had been privy to twenty years ago. She worried about birth defects and was especially apprehensive about the possibility of her children having Down's Syndrome as a result of her memories of her own younger sister's affliction with it.

When Marianne had her first son, she was thirty years old. She felt that her scoliosis curves progressed with this pregnancy because, though she still felt no pain, her back seemed visually worse than it had been before. Of course Marianne did not mind this; she was preoccupied with the birth of her beautiful son.

"We were so thrilled to have a child at that point in life because we were older," explains Marianne. "We were so thrilled with him."

Soon after the birth of their son, Marianne's husband was tranferred to Dayton, Ohio. Marianne quit her job in teaching and administration to devote all her time to being a mother. Then, six months after the young family had moved to Ohio, tragedy struck.

At nineteen months old, Marianne's son was diagnosed with neuroblastoma, a cancer of the systemic nervous system that occurs in babies. Marianne and her son temporarily relocated to Sloan Kettering Hospital in New York, while Marianne's husband alternated between his work in Ohio and his family in New York.

"My son and I essentially lived there [at the hospital], and I carried him up and down those halls endlessly," Marianne remembers. "I could tell that carrying him so much was really making my curvature worse, but it didn't matter at that point." Marianne's son died when he was twenty-six months old. Just six weeks later, her daughter was born.

"At the time of my son's diagnosis, I was already pregnant with my daughter, which was really a blessing, because I don't think I would have ever opened myself up to that kind of pain again," Marianne admits.

After the death of their first son and the birth of their daughter, Marianne and her husband decided that they wanted to have another child. Marianne was thirty-four years old, and she knew that she would have to do something about her scoliosis in the future. Therefore, she felt that if she was going to have another child, she had to do it right away. Fifteen months after the birth of her daughter, Marianne gave birth to her second son. During her pregnancies, Marianne's scoliosis curves were hovering around sixty-four degrees in the thoracic region and sixty-five degrees in the lumbar region.

Following her pregnancies, Marianne began to inquire about a family history of scoliosis. She was concerned about her own case of the disorder as well as her children's potential to demonstrate spinal curvature in the future. She found out that she did have a relatively strong family history of scoliosis and that no one in her family had really known about their scoliosis until Marianne had been diagnosed back in 1960. Marianne learned that a few of her cousins have scoliosis, but none of their cases had become as severe as hers.

As soon as her second son was old enough to walk, Marianne decided to have the spinal fusion she had been postponing for so many years. First, she visited a scoliosis surgeon in Miami. Getting to know this surgeon, Marianne realized that she did not have the right feeling about him.

"I think that you connect—you either feel it's right or it's not right," Marianne explains. Luckily, Marianne found a doctor she really liked on her second try. "The minute I saw him, I felt comfortable with him." This second surgeon proposed a French surgical method that was new at the time, called the Cotrel procedure. Liking her surgeon and trusting him to make the correct judgment calls concerning her surgery, Marianne agreed to have the Cotrel procedure.

Marianne had a spinal fusion in 1985; she was thirty-eight years old at the time, and her curves measured seventy-two degrees in the thoracic region and sixty degrees in the lumbar region.

Pre-operatively, Marianne's husband took measures at home to prepare their children, who were ages four and two at the time, for their mother's surgery.

"I'll never forget that my husband had made a doll," Marianne says. "He took one of the kids' dolls, and he put patches on the back of the doll and drew on the back of the doll what they [the surgeons] would be doing to me so that they [the children] would see. It was interesting for the kids; it was a very visual thing. They understood what was happening and what my limitations would be when I came back from the hospital—I couldn't pick them up, and all that."

In preparing herself for the surgery, Marianne visited a music therapist at a local children's hospital. This therapist taught Marianne how to transcend pain through music, and Marianne felt that the therapy was greatly effective. She was able to use a lot less medication than most people do after surgery. Even after she returned home from the hospital, Marianne could listen to music to make the pain go away. Interestingly, any pain that Marianne could not ward off by way of music therapy she welcomed.

In addition to having the instrumentation implanted into her spine, Marianne wanted to have her rib hump cut out—mainly for cosmetic reasons. "My doctor told me that there was a chance that I would have a punctured lung if he cut my rib hump, but I still agreed to it," Marianne says. "I didn't care. I wanted it [my rib hump] cut. I did end up having a punctured lung, but it didn't really bother me that much. The recovery was wonderful. It went well. Nothing happened."

Virtually Marianne's entire spine was fused; bone graft from her hip was used to complete the fusion. Post-operatively, she had neither a brace nor a cast, and she began teaching part-time at a community college within one month following her surgery. Since she had her spinal fusion in 1985, Marianne has done everything from raising children to rollerblading to skiing and has yet to experience a single problem with her spine.

Today, Marianne maintains an active lifestyle and performs aerobics every day to keep in shape and to maintain flexibility.

Despite the fact that her surgeon cut her rib hump in hopes of abolishing any visible physical deformity, Marianne still has a slight hump in the right thoracic region of her back. She is very comfortable talking about it and was happy to show me that, thirteen years after surgery, her hump—though diminished and much less noticeable—is still present. Though she is careful about buying clothes that camouflage her slight deformity, Marianne is neither embarrassed nor hindered by her scoliosis—and she never has been.

Marianne has, with the help of a strong husband and family, withstood all that life has presented her—both good and bad. Marianne is busy raising her two teenagers, neither of whom has scoliosis and both of whom she is infinitely proud of and grateful for.

"They do not have it [scoliosis]," Marianne says. "They've been screened carefully. I am very, very grateful . . . my children are special gifts, and I feel very blessed to have them."

JANICE
"I was ignorant of my curve."

Throughout her life, Janice has been no stranger to deformity. When she was a child, her mother had a chest deformity that earned her the nickname "chicken breast." Her father had "what looked like scoliosis," though the definite cause of his deformity was never revealed. Janice's older sister had a mild case of scoliosis, and her younger sister would later find out that she, too, had the disorder. In 1950, when she was thirteen years old, Janice began to exhibit scoliosis in her own spine.

Janice was diagnosed with scoliosis through a school screening program, yet in 1950 school screening programs for scoliosis were few and far between. She went to one of the few schools where the students *were* checked for scoliosis. At the time of Janice's diagnosis, there were few treatment options open to people with mild curves. She was told by doctors that observation of her curve would be treatment enough until it progressed to a more significant degree. Of course Janice believed what she was told, left the doctor's office, and carried on with her busy teenage life.

Janice's scoliosis got her excused from many gym activities, including using the "horse apparatus," and inhibited her from making the cheerleading squad—this was a real disappointment. However, she remained active in many sports and was a majorette in her school's marching band. Janice also played the piano. She played for hours each day, sharpening her skills, and eventually won contests and music scholarships. She describes herself as having been "a skinny kid" and

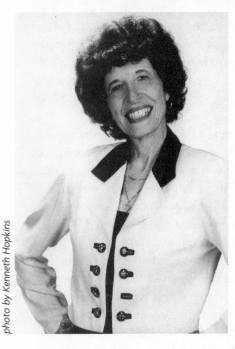

photo by Kenneth Hopkins

remembers having an oddly shaped body with "no waist." Therefore, Janice—unlike most girls her age—was usually quite deterred from going clothes shopping.

By the time she was seventeen, Janice's thoracic scoliosis curve had progressed to measure a substantial thirty degrees; the degree measure of her lumbar curve at the time (which had formed *as a result* of the thoracic curve—to balance it) was unknown. At this point, doctors recommended that she hang upside down from a bar to stretch and straighten her spine. In the midst of her doing this bar-hanging, Janice traveled to New York City upon the recommendation of her family physician. She saw an orthopedic doctor there who shocked her by recommending surgery. At that time, scoliosis surgeries were done without instrumentation. The spine was straightened and fused independent of any rod system; the catch was that the patient was immobile for one year following the surgery. When Janice heard that having surgery would require her to lay flat on her back for one year, she immediately refused. She was active in theater, singing, and dancing at the time and could not have imagined giving up any of her activities.

"I said, 'no way,'" Janice remembers.

"If you don't have surgery, your scoliosis will interfere with your spinal cord, and you will become paralyzed," her doctor told her.

"Thank you very much, but I'll take my chances," responded Janice. "I was ignorant of my curve," she reflects now.

After she visited this doctor, Janice returned to high school and obtained her degree. She experienced many illnesses—most of them bronchial—throughout the next few years. As she turned eighteen and then nineteen years old, Janice began to see a hump in her back. Her friends never told her that her back was crooked, but she began to see it herself; and it really bothered her. Despite her deformity and her embarrassment, Janice got married at the age of nineteen. After she married, she went to college; after college, she gave birth to two baby girls (within a few years of one another). During this time, Janice's scoliosis was progressing at a rate of one to two degrees per year, though she "pretty much forgot about it" for the next few decades.

"Everything started to happen when I was forty-four," she remembers. Janice went to an orthopedic specialist in New York because of some hip discomfort she had been having. After X rays had been taken, this doctor was more concerned with Janice's spine than he was with her hips. He told Janice that she had "wedge-shaped" vertebrae; they were very rigid and, although they needed surgery, he could not do it. The case was too difficult for this doctor, and he feared the risk of paralysis. He recommended doctors in Hong Kong, Paris, and Minneapolis who, at the time, were the leaders in scoliosis surgery.

In search of a doctor who *would* attempt to correct her scoliosis but hesitant to start looking in Hong Kong, Paris, or Minneapolis, Janice got a second opinion from another doctor in New York. This doctor said that he would have her lie down and do a halo stretch in traction (pulling Janice up from a metal halo around her head and down from her hips) for three weeks before he would operate. Janice simply did not like this idea; she thought it sounded dangerous and slightly barbaric. She therefore sought a third opinion. This time, Janice traveled from her home in Florida to Minneapolis, where she saw an expert in scoliosis surgery. It was at this visit that Janice found the surgeon whom she would ultimately choose.

At first, Janice really disliked this surgeon. She found him to be "very defensive"—he was not used to having patients with long lists of questions. When Janice asked him about the previously recommended traction, he said, "No way!" He told Janice that traction would most likely cause an injury to her spinal cord. Relieved that she had sought a third opinion before she had gone into traction, she continued to ask questions. The two bantered back and forth for their entire first encounter and, in Janice's words, "did not hit it off." Janice now tells people, "Do not judge a doctor by your first visit."

"Sometimes you are not listening to the doctor's answers," she explains. "You may be presenting yourself in a way that may not correctly represent your real objective. You may be tense and angry. So give the doctor another chance, or call back and present your questions in written form so that he or she has a chance to see your questions before your next appointment."

Despite the tension between Janice and this newfound specialist, this doctor said that he would be willing to perform the surgery. He suggested a plain, posterior fusion and straightening of the thoracic curve only. This doctor would choose not to touch Janice's lumbar curve because, on Janice's bending films, the lumbar curve had straightened out almost completely. In other words, since Janice's lumbar curve was flexible enough to self-correct when she bent over, it was presumably flexible enough to be trusted to straighten on its own once the thoracic curve that had caused it had been surgically straightened.

After her visit with the doctor in Minneapolis, Janice's attitude was, "No way would I use him!" The way she saw it, she had two conflicting opinions from two doctors—the second and third ones she had seen; the first doctor had not really given Janice an opinion. Not knowing what to do or who to listen to, Janice decided to do some independent investigation. She and her husband, Stanley, went to the library and started their research. They obtained medical journals and read literature; they found as much information as they could and extracted from it what valuable information pertained to Janice's particular case. Interestingly, what Janice and Stanley found was that ninety percent of the available articles on scoliosis were *from* Minneapolis. Most of the articles had been written by surgeons at the hospital in Minneapolis, and many had been written by the surgeon Janice had seen just a few weeks before. It was at this point that Janice and Stanley knew in their hearts that the opinion of the doctor in Minneapolis had been the right one. Feeling as though they had done enough research, Janice and Stanley closed the books, got on the phone, and made an appointment for Janice's surgery.

Pre-operatively, Janice began to exhibit a lot of unexpected behavioral anxiety. Most vividly, she remembers that, while she and Stanley were shopping for a car one day, she "got upset, threw a cup in the air, and drove down the road hysterical." Throughout this difficult period, Stanley was very supportive of Janice. He suggested that she see a psychiatrist to help her cope better with the prospect of surgery. Janice took Stanley's suggestion and began to see a psychiatrist—a decision she grew to embrace. Though the psychiatrist did not know anything about scoliosis, Janice taught him. It would turn out that Janice's psychiatrist would call her on the night before she had surgery (and on all of the "nights before surgery" that Janice would end up enduring throughout the next several years) to work through her anxiety. Even if he was on vacation, the psychiatrist would call Janice. Janice feels that this man was very salutary for her mental well-being and an integral part of her getting through surgery.

Janice arrived in Minneapolis the day before her surgery and was admitted to the hospital. (Today, patients are generally admitted to hospitals on the day of surgery.) She met with the nursing team who would be treating her and had her pre-operative X rays taken. Janice had already given three units of blood at a hospital near her home in Florida in preparation for the surgery. Between that time and the day before the surgery, Janice's former weight of 127 pounds had dwindled to a mere 102 pounds, which meagerly draped her five-foot, three-inch frame. She lost her appetite, resulting in a loss of twenty-five pounds. She would regret this after her surgery, when she would feel weak and fragile.

The night before her surgery, Janice's doctor came into her hospital room to visit her.

"I never thought I'd see you again," he said, alluding to their originally antagonistic relationship.

"You don't know me very well," she responded. "I did my homework, and you're the one!"

In July 1982, Janice's eighty-six-degree lumbar curve was surgically corrected to fifty-eight degrees; her sixty-nine-degree lumbar curve then straightened on its own to forty-seven degrees. The fusion was done with Harrington rod instrumentation contoured to Janice's spine. After the surgery, Janice woke up frightened and in excruciating pain. She found that the doctor, who had planned to remove one of her ribs to decrease the obvious hump in her back, had ended up removing portions of seven of her ribs. The ribs are made of cartilage and do grow back, but they do not grow back with the same strength as normal ribs. Therefore, by cutting the ribs and allowing them to grow back softer and less prominent, doctors can actually decrease the heights and perceptibility of scoliosis-related rib humps. In retrospect, Janice attributes the present slightness of her rib hump to her doctor's decision to perform an unexpected thoracoplasty. Though the cutting of her ribs gave her a lot of post-operative pain, Janice says that her doctor did a "beautiful job" and that she is glad he cut her ribs and improved her cosmetic appearance. As Janice was just waking up from her anesthesia-induced sleep and feeling that unexpected pain in her ribs, her tired eyes discerned the face of the surgeon who had assisted during her surgery. This surgeon was sitting at Janice's bedside in the recovery room.

"I think we should have fused your lumbar region, too," he admitted to her. "We didn't do it because you felt corrected on the [operating] table—let's see what happens." In other words, while the doctors treating Janice had thought that her lumbar curve would correct on its own once the thoracic curve had been corrected, they had been wrong. Though Janice's lumbar curve had straightened a bit on its own, it had not straightened as considerably as the doctors had hoped. And there was no telling whether Janice's lumbar curve would now start to progress again, seeing as it was not fused but, rather, free to move as it pleased. As it turned out, the assistant surgeon was right, but Janice would not deal with the lumbar section of her spine for quite a while.

Following her surgery, Janice lay flat for ten days. After these ten days began her calamitous road to a marginal recovery. After having lain in bed for ten days, Janice was casted very tightly. When she finally stood up, she noticed that her cast was crooked, so the cast had to be redone. One can imagine the pain involved in being rolled around and fitted for a body cast just days after having a spinal fusion. Even the second body cast did not fit Janice very well. She lost weight and learned to deal with pain on a daily basis. Because of the difficulty Janice was having with her body cast, a few weeks after surgery the hospital staff put her into a back brace. The brace, like the cast, was poorly fitted; but at least it was removable. Janice wore the brace all the time except for the fifteen minutes every day during which she showered.

For the next several weeks, Janice stayed near her hospital in Minneapolis. She and Stanley had rented an apartment there before the surgery because they had known that Janice would need to visit her doctor post-operatively and that the trip home from Minnesota to Florida (and subsequent trips back for check-ups) would be difficult and expensive. During her stay in Minneapolis, Janice walked three miles each day. She wore her back brace while she walked around the many lakes and malls in the Minneapolis area.

"It was wonderful," Janice says of her stay in Minnesota. Once she had been discharged from the hospital and had begun nonstrenuous exercise (walking) and functioning on her own, Janice recovered quickly. Her surgery had taken place in July, and by the end of August, she was ready to go home. Janice flew from Minnesota to Florida while Stanley drove home.

By November of that year, Janice was "in agony" from her brace. She had developed sores on her body as a result of the brace rubbing against her skin and was miserably uncomfortable. She returned to Minneapolis and "threw the brace at them [the hospital staff]." Janice's doctor saw by the sores on her body that she was right about her brace; he had a new brace made for Janice immediately. The new brace was much more comfortable than the old one had been. However, during the six months following this visit to Minneapolis, Janice found that she was bending in her brace. Her lumbar curve, which had not been fused, had, unfortunately, continued to progress. Janice's body was bending so much that it actually began to bend her brace and eventually made a hole in it. So, after eight months in this second brace, Janice stopped wearing it. She returned, once again, to Minnesota, for she knew that she would have to make plans for additional surgery.

In July 1983, Janice found herself in Minnesota once again. For this surgery, Janice's doctor would fuse the lumbar part of her spine all the way to the sacrum to complete the job he had begun one year ago. In days prior to the surgery, Janice had thought that it would be an anterior surgery. The night before her surgery, she was informed that the fusion of her lumbar spine would require both an anterior and a posterior approach. The next day, while Janice was on the operating table during the anterior component of this second surgery, a tornado ripped through Minnesota. The tornado wiped out the hospital's electricity, and Janice's doctors were left operating on her for twelve hours via a generator. Following the surgery, Janice lay in bed for two weeks. Then it was time for her doctor to perform the posterior part of the surgery. This posterior component of Janice's lumbar fusion was technically her third surgery in a series of many. (Today an anterior/posterior surgery is regarded as one surgery and is usually performed in a single operating session.)

During her recuperation, Janice walked around Minnesota's lakes and malls once again. Janice did run into a bit of trouble with recovery this time; her doctor told her that she should have eaten more and exercised more before the surgery. Being in good shape ensures an easier, faster recovery. Having learned an invaluable lesson, Janice now emphasizes the importance of a proper diet and exercise presurgically. Janice also recommends biofeedback[22] before and after surgery. "Taking biofeedback is one of the best things you can do presurgically," Janice says.

Janice had also "learned how to breathe" and made a special relaxation tape. Her nurses were amazed at how these strategies lessened Janice's need for post-operative medication.

Following the fusion of her lumbar spine, Janice found that she was very uncomfortable. She was thin at the time and saw that the rods in her spine were too close to her skin; they were almost visible. When she complained to her doctor about her rods, he agreed that they were creating unnecessary problems and decided to remove them. Thus, Janice returned to Minneapolis for her fourth surgery just eighteen months after she had undergone her third. This time, the surgery was less complicated; she just had her rods removed.

Three months after the removal of her rods, Janice decided to get her body back into shape. One day, she went to the local YMCA in Florida to do some carefully supervised stretching exercises. The next day, she felt "excruciating pain." Janice was unable to sit back or to lie in the car. She would scream if the car hit a bump. At a scoliosis conference soon after, she happened to meet with some doctors who looked at her and said, "Your stomach is sticking out; get an X ray immediately."

Janice then went to a local doctor, desperate to have X rays taken and to see what was wrong with her. At the doctor's office, Janice was in so much pain that she could barely get on the X-ray table. The X rays showed that a remaining wire (from the instrumentation that had been removed) in her spine had cut her at the junction of her T8 and T9 vertebrae. To remove all of the wires involved in the particular instrumentation system Janice had had in her spine was impossible; therefore, when her doctor had removed her rods three months ago, he had not removed the wire between Janice's T8 and T9 vertebrae. The doctor would not have left this wire in if he could have helped it, but he had been unable to remove it. The remaining wire had not caused Janice any problems until she had exercised that one day. Now, she was in chronic, excruciating pain. The day after she had obtained those very telling X rays in Florida, Janice called her doctor in Minnesota and said, "I'm coming up!"

Janice's fifth surgery, which occurred in 1985, was, thus, a real emergency. Janice and Stanley immediately flew to Minnesota for the occasion. Traveling from the temperate Florida weather to the freezing cold Minnesota winter was unpleasant for Janice, as was traveling in general because she was in so much pain. Once she had arrived in Minneapolis, she was on the operating table in no time. Her fifth surgery consisted of the anterior replacement of the troublesome wire with new instrumentation. A few days after this surgery, Janice went in for her sixth surgery, which was the posterior portion of inserting this new instrumentation and creating a new fusion.

Eighteen months later, in 1987, Janice returned for the last time to Minneapolis to have her rods removed. In three to four days after her second rod removal—and her seventh surgery—Janice felt recovered and ready to go home. With years of seasoning and experience under her belt, Janice had become an "old pro" at having surgery.

Today, Janice is a wife, a mother, and a grandmother. Janice's two daughters—one of whom has two children—have both grown and married. One daughter has a slight scoliosis curve that never required treatment; the other shows no signs of scoliosis. Two of Janice's nieces have scoliosis; one has a sixty-degree curve and is planning to have surgery soon. Though Janice has not had any scoliosis surgeries in the past eleven years, she remains keenly aware and careful of her body and her scoliosis. She and Stanley spend their days running a national support and information organization for people with scoliosis, planning fundraisers for scoliosis research, and using their experience in dealing with this disorder to help others.

Looking at Janice, it is hard to believe that beneath the well-dressed, active exterior lies a woman who lives every day of her life with pain. The numerous surgeries Janice has undergone have left her limited in motion and unable to bend straight over from her hips. Despite this, Janice would *never* think of herself as being handicapped. She only thinks of how appreciative she is for her "wonderful cosmetic correction" and maintains that she is happy to have endured what she did.

"I'm grateful," she says. "I'm sorry I didn't do it younger. I really am."

Author's Note: *During the time when Janice was in her post-surgical brace, she founded a scoliosis support and information group in Palm Beach County. Her group's first meeting occurred in February 1983. Janice was president of her Palm Beach County support organization for twelve years before she became the president of a national organization that provides support and information for people with scoliosis.*

Advice from a Person Who Has Been through It All

• Know who your anesthesiologist is.
• Do not judge a doctor on the basis of your first visit.

- Do research on your own; make decisions for yourself.
- Always get your operative report from the surgery. You are entitled to it.
- Your hospital is important. Your aftercare is important. Choose these carefully.
- The post-surgical care is as important as the surgery. Make sure you go into the Intensive Care Unit for at least a day before you are transferred into a regular room—even if the hospital tries to deny you ICU care.
- Pre-operative and post-operative nutrition is very important. Make sure that you are consuming enough calories and that you are eating and drinking the right foods and beverages.
- Try to exercise prior to surgery; the better shape you are in, the faster your recovery will be.
- If you are an adult (especially one living alone), make sure you go through occupational therapy before you leave the hospital. In other words, post-operatively, you should know how to brush your teeth without bending over the sink and how to move so that you do not stretch your spine, etc.
- Try biofeedback, both pre- and post-operatively.
- Many hospitals today are short-staffed. Be sure that, during your stay, your sheets are cleaned every day. This is important to prevent things such as staph infections. There is no such thing as an environment that is too clean; remember that some people are more prone to staph (infections) than others are.

LINDA

Battling Adolescent "Humiliation" And Emerging As Victor

In 1955, a pediatrician appeared at Linda's home; he had come to examine Linda's brother, who had been mildly ill. What the pediatrician seemed to be more concerned about, though, was the protruding shoulder blade he noticed in twelve-year-old Linda's back. He informed Linda's mother that her daughter's spine may be curved and recommended that she take Linda to see an orthopedic surgeon.

Linda and her mother were already quite familiar with the hospital at this point. Linda had had patent ductus arteriosis (a heart defect) as a baby. Though she had not had any complications or difficulties with her heart after this defect had been corrected, Linda had been followed by a doctor at the hospital's pediatric cardiac clinic throughout her childhood.

An orthopedic surgeon at the hospital confirmed that Linda had scoliosis. This diagnosis, however, did not come as a shock to either Linda or her mother because scoliosis ran in their family. Linda's eighty-seven-year-old paternal grandmother had a severe, untreated "S" curve and had lived most of her life with boundless energy and no problems. Linda's family had been under the impression that scoliosis was the cause of nothing more than physical deformity. They had no idea of the health implications of some scoliosis curves and did not imagine ever having to treat Linda's curve any more than they had seen her grandmother's curve treated.

Upon Linda's diagnosis, her grandmother insisted that she see the chiropractor that she, herself, had been seeing for a number of years. Linda went to this chiropractor for a full year. And, while the chiropractic treatment did loosen her spine up a bit, it did not do anything to correct or to treat her scoliosis. In fact, the chiropractor said honestly to Linda's mother, "I cannot treat this child. She has to be treated by an orthopedic doctor."

Therefore, an orthopedic doctor followed Linda's scoliosis for the next couple of years. Treated with observation alone, Linda almost entirely forgot about her scoliosis and got very involved in a number of physical activities. During her early teenage years, she became serious about ballet, tap dance, and ice skating. Her acumen in each of these activities sharpened, and she came to enjoy them more every day.

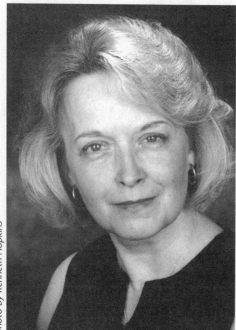

photo by Kenneth Hopkins

"But just as I became serious about my lessons," Linda says, "I heard the word surgery." At fourteen, Linda was told by her orthopedic surgeon—who had been observing her scoliosis for two years—that surgery was now in order. This reality struck Linda with herculean force. She describes herself as

having been "speechless" and "devastated." Upon hearing that she needed to have surgery, Linda visited with her cardiologist, seeking in him
both emotional support and information. She wanted to know how her
scoliosis would affect her if it went untreated, whether surgery was
really necessary. And although Linda's cardiologist wanted to protect
her feelings, he was not about to lie to her. With Linda's best health
interests in mind, the cardiologist admitted to Linda that, if she left her
scoliosis untreated, it would progress to such a degree that it would
eventually rotate her ribs and put pressure on her lungs and heart. This
promise foreboded a dangerous situation in Linda's case, for her heart
was already less strong than most other hearts. Though Linda dreaded
having any sort of surgery and giving up the activities she had come to
love so much, she did not want to jeopardize her health. Therefore,
Linda hesitantly decided that it would be in her best interest to undergo the scoliosis surgery.

Six weeks before her scheduled surgery date, Linda went to the hospital's scoliosis clinic for a pre-admission examination. She recalls that
this examination was a "very humiliating experience." The nurse who
escorted her to the examination, as well as the doctors who performed
the examination, showed very little concern for Linda's fragile adolescent
emotions. At fourteen years old, Linda was asked to strip down into a
bikini and to cover herself with a hospital gown. Once she had changed,
she was presented to a group of twenty doctors and related health professionals who sat waiting in a classroom. As Linda entered the doctor-
filled room, the nurse whipped the hospital gown off her small body
without warning. Linda stood almost completely bare in the middle of
the large, unfamiliar room as the twenty doctors and health professionals "checked" her. They observed Linda's body; asked her to bend and
stretch every which way; stood up and encircled her to see her more
closely; touched her back where it was curved; and recorded notes on
what they observed. Linda's parents had received no word of what this
so-called pre-admission examination would entail. They had left Linda at
the hospital under the impression that she would be in good hands.
Unfortunately, Linda found herself struggling in a sea of cold, unfriendly
medical experts. There was nothing she could do to stop them, and what
they did to her left behind painful memories of humiliation and deep-
seated emotional scars that would last a lifetime. Today, this sort of
treatment would be considered an insensitive violation of privacy bor-
dering on child abuse. In 1957, it was common practice.

The protocol for surgery in 1957 not only included the pre-admission examination, but it included a pre-operative casting procedure. Following her examination, Linda was taken to a room known to the hospital personnel as the plaster room—and known to the patients as the "torture chamber." Over the next six weeks, Linda was put into a series of casts. The first cast extended from her shoulders to her hips. After that cast had been applied, a collar-type attachment was added to it. The purpose of this casting process was to prepare Linda for the traction that she would endure continually for the six weeks leading up to her surgery.

The traction procedure involved Linda being given a sedative and then placed on a traction table for hours at a time. Nurses attached devices on this special table to the shoulder and hip portions of Linda's cast. Pulling up on Linda's shoulders and down on her hips, the table applied much force to Linda's spine. This procedure was done in an effort to stretch the spine and to see what degree of correction would be possible to achieve during surgery. The more limber the spine was forced to be, the better correction doctors felt they could achieve. Traction is a treatment method no longer used today because it was later found to be minimally effective and deemed to be barbaric and inhuman. Unfortunately for Linda, traction was an accepted mode of treatment for scoliosis during the time when she was being treated. Like most nightmares, memories of being in traction continue to linger in the minds of those who endured it. Though Linda is now an adult, a wife, and a mother of grown children, visions and sensations of the rudimentary scoliosis treatment she endured as a fourteen-year-old still haunt her.

On December 20, 1957, surgeons operated on Linda for four hours, fusing her spine from the T5 vertebra to the L1 vertebra and changing her sixty-eight degree thoracic curve to a twenty-eight degree curve. The doctors took an old-fashioned approach Linda's surgery and used no instrumentation—*after all, instrumentation was still relatively new at that time.* They simply made the posterior incision, straightened the spine by way of force, and applied bone graft from the hospital's tissue bank to Linda's spine in order to make it fuse in that straight position. The day of the surgery, Linda was under heavy anesthesia and experienced no pain. When she woke the next morning, though, she experienced severe pain. Her doctors and nurses relaxed her with narcotics while they molded her post-operative body cast—which was much like her pre-operative cast—and made her lie in bed for a full week. Linda remembers that Christmas (five days after her surgery) as being particularly awful.

Linda was left to function in her post-operative body cast for the next three months. She was monitored closely by nurses and assisted frequently by a physical therapist. Once she was standing again, Linda was happy to realize that she had grown two inches when her spine had been straightened. This was the favorable aspect of the surgery.

For a total of four-and-a-half months (six weeks before surgery and three months after surgery) Linda lived in a body cast and resided amongst hospital workers and fellow patients in the pediatric ward of the hospital. The social climate there was odd. Linda remembers there being a tremendous camaraderie among the scoliosis patients; she saw patients whose cases were worse than her own and was, therefore, able to feel better about herself. The many young scoliosis patients in that hospital supported one another throughout the different stages of one another's surgeries. For that four-and-a-half-month period, Linda found a sort of comfort in a makeshift family of doctors, nurses, and ailing children. The only glimpses Linda got of a real family during her stay at the hospital occurred when her mother visited her once or twice each week and on weekends (the hospital was over an hour away—by car— from Linda's home). Sometimes, Linda's mother would bring Linda's cats along with her and would put them up to the hospital window—animals were not allowed in the hospital—so that Linda could visit with them.

Not only did the hospital function as Linda's home for the four-and-a-half-month period, but it functioned as her school and her recreational ground. Linda participated in a full school program at the hospital, with teachers, a principal, and fellow patients who were students. In terms of recreational opportunities, the hospital offered movies every Saturday night, ran "wheelchair games," and hired entertainers for the kids. Linda remembers seeing Brenda Lee, a child entertainer at the time, perform.

The hospital was not just a place for friendships, fun, and games, though. It was a place where Linda had to struggle toward her recovery and endure the humiliation of being an adolescent in a body cast. When Linda had first arrived at the hospital and was put into her body cast, she had noticed that all the patients in the pediatric scoliosis ward had the same haircut. The nurses wanted to cut Linda's hair to make wearing the body cast easier—and their own jobs easier, too. By cutting the patients' hair, they avoided having to wash it frequently, having to comb it, and having to fuss with it. Nevertheless, Linda would not let the nurses cut her hair. A year after Linda had set this precedent, all the girls in the pediatric scoliosis ward had ponytails.

Two months after her surgery, Linda started sitting and then walking with the help of parallel bars. Soon she was able to walk with just crutches. During the time that she was in the cast, Linda experienced immense physical difficulty; the cast was so heavy that it made her unable to walk or move very easily. Because of atrophied muscles and a loss of appetite, Linda lost about twenty pounds while she was in her cast. And throughout the year that she was in the cast (she wore it for six more months after she returned home from the hospital), she and her fellow castwearers were referred to as "penguins" because of the difficulty they had walking.

Linda was finally discharged from the hospital on March 17, 1958. By that time, she was able to walk on her own, despite her being in a body cast, and was off all pain medication. She was able to sit in the car for the ride home because her parents had situated her comfortably, yet she was not able to return to school once she arrived at home because she felt that the forty-five minute bus ride to and from school would be too painful and uncomfortable to endure. Instead of going to school, Linda would have a homebound tutor come to her house five days a week.

Ten and a half months after her surgery, Linda had her cast removed. The body the cast had covered for so long was now marred by ulcerations—primarily under the arms and on the hips. These scars would last for years. One year after her surgery, Linda returned to the hospital for a followup appointment. Doctors determined that her fusion had held and that she would not have to return to the hospital for another ten years. At her ten-year followup appointment, Linda, now age twenty-four, demonstrated a minimal loss of correction; her previously twenty-eight degree curve had moved to thirty-two degrees.

Linda went on to graduate from high school and from college. She got married and became pregnant twice. Neither pregnancy presented her with any back problems and both her babies were delivered via cesarean sections. After her childhood, Linda never again thought about her scoliosis and was never affected by it—with the exception, perhaps, of occasional fatigue in her right flank muscle.

At the age of forty-five, Linda was broadsided in a car accident and, afterwards, began to experience intensifying back pain. In addition to the pain, Linda began to notice a gradual decrease in her height. A routine bone density scan done by her primary care physician showed Linda that she had "the bones of a twenty-two year old" and ascertained that the pain Linda was experiencing was not related to osteoporosis. However, Linda was still concerned about her spine. Her physician therefore encouraged her to see an orthopedic doctor to follow up on her scoliosis history. After searching on the Internet, seeking personal references, and attending local scoliosis support group meetings, Linda found a doctor she wished to visit. Her examination with this doctor showed that her fusion had remained solid but that she had lost her correction of curvature. In other words, even though Linda's spine was still strong, fused, and unbroken, the fusion without the instrumentation had not been enough to hold her spine straight for a long period of time. The spine that was virtually straight after the surgery in 1987 had now sunken back into a curved position. Linda's original thoracic curve, which she had last known to measure thirty-two degrees, had progressed to fifty degrees. In addition to the thoracic curve, Linda now had a fifty-five-degree lumbar curve that had developed naturally to counterbalance the thoracic curve.

Despite his findings, the doctor Linda had gone to told her that she was not a surgical candidate. To have any sort of corrective surgery at this age would be a risk not worth taking for Linda. She functions well and appears to be balanced despite the curvature of her spine; having surgery as a mature adult would potentially present her with more physical problems than she has now. To cope with her scoliosis as an adult who is not a surgical candidate, Linda exercises and swims. She also attends monthly meetings of a scoliosis support group in her area in order to keep abreast of the latest in scoliosis treatments, developments, and research.

Author's Note: *Many teenagers today view surgery as a terrible fate. It is easy to think of yourself as the victim of scoliosis and to approach your surgery as if it is the worst possible thing that could be happening to you. I know this because I viewed scoliosis surgery as being a horribly painful and difficult procedure until Linda shared her story with me. In comparison with the barbaric, traumatizing surgical techniques used when Linda had surgery, the surgical techniques of today seem relatively simple and easy. In just forty years, year-long stints in body casts have dissolved into no use of body casts; four-month-long stays in the* *hospital have dwindled to five day-long stays; and surgeries that left major physical and emotional scars have become surgeries that quickly and easily bring health and straight spines. Considering this, who knows what surgical techniques might be like just a few years from now? I admire Linda for persevering through an experience that most people today are unable even to imagine. Her determination through her battle with scoliosis and her motivation to go on and live a normal life after having been through so much pain is truly amazing. Linda's story has made me realize that, since I have to be afflicted with scoliosis, I am lucky to be afflicted with it today rather than forty years ago.*

ALISON
"Turtle"

Among the acres of horse farms in the northern part of Florida lives thirty-year-old Alison with her husband, her son, and her horse. When she is not busy tending to Kyle, her two-year-old, or training her thoroughbred, Alison works as a target case manager, linking children with psychiatric and/or medical services. Presently, she is working with juvenile delinquents ranging from age thirteen to nineteen. Upon meeting Alison, anyone would be able to tell that she was the smart, popular, cheerleader "type" in high school. What most people are not able to tell however, is that throughout Alison's high school years of friends, fun, and cheerleading, she was dealing with scoliosis. In fact, Alison had a scoliosis surgery each year throughout her four years in high school, earning her the nickname "Turtle" because she was, as she puts it, "always in a shell"—a body cast. Each day that passes, Alison's bout with scoliosis becomes less of a reality and more of a memory. But Alison is positive that she will never forget about her years of surgeries and "shells"; she even collects turtle knickknacks to make sure that she will remember.

Nineteen years ago, when Alison was eleven years old, her mother took her to the pediatrician because of an ear infection. At that visit, the pediatrician happened to notice a protrusion of one side of Alison's back. Examining her back more closely, the pediatrician discerned that Alison had scoliosis. After he had diagnosed Alison, the pediatrician proceeded to say that he would just need to "observe" her scoliosis until it progressed to a degree that required treatment. Not knowing any better than to trust what their doctor was saying, Alison and her mother agreed that Alison would be observed and returned home, bare-

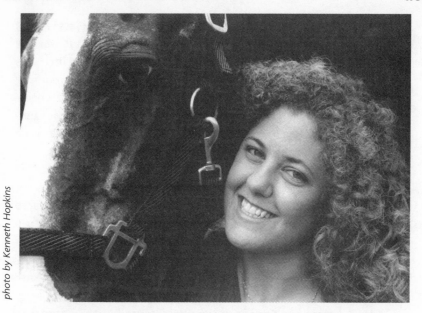

photo by Kenneth Hopkins

ly remembering that Alison had just been diagnosed with anything.

In the next few years, Alison became an avid horseback rider, as well as a devoted dancer. In eighth grade, Alison made the cheerleading squad at her middle school. She was still busy learning new cheers when, in 1981, she was abruptly told by her pediatrician that her scoliosis now required surgery. Alison's and her family's immediate reaction to this news was devastation. Then, as Allison thought about having to give up horseback riding, dancing, and cheerleading, she simply said that she would not have the surgery. Eventually, though, Alison's doctor—who knew that the rotation and curvature of her spine would begin to affect her health if she did not have surgery—convinced Alison's family that surgery was unarguably necessary. Alison's family then convinced fourteen-year-old Alison to have surgery by telling her that it would not change any aspect of her life. After the surgery, they told her, she could go back to horseback riding, dancing, and cheerleading—though they had no idea whether their claims were true. Nevertheless, Alison believed her family, trusted her doctor, and agreed to have the surgery.

Alison and her family had not thought about Alison's scoliosis very much at this point. They had never imagined that it would require surgery, did not know what the surgery entailed, had no idea how long the surgery and recovery would take, and were altogether poorly informed as to scoliosis and its implications. Nevertheless, Alison would have the surgery because her doctor had told her it was the right thing to do—and she had made up her mind not to let it change her life or her attitude. Before *and* after surgery, Alison would be determined to continue with horseback riding, dancing, and cheerleading. Her positive attitude would infiltrate her entire surgical experience, and the strength she maintained would make the experience bearable for her otherwise distressed family.

Surgery #1: Before Freshman Year: For three weeks before her surgery, Alison wore a body cast. Her doctor felt that Alison's wearing a tailored body cast (much like a back brace) would force her spine into a straighter position, thereby making it more stretchable and flexible for the surgery. It was hoped that this would aid the doctor during surgery to force Alison's spine into a straighter position and achieve a greater correction of her scoliosis.

The day before her surgery, Alison was admitted to the hospital to have her body cast cut off. The next morning, she was in surgery for nine hours. Alison's doctor inserted twelve-inch-long Harrington rods into the tiny spine of four-foot, eleven-inch-tall Alison. After the surgery, Alison would find that she had grown to five feet, one and a half inches. She would not stand up, though, for several days after her surgery.

During her ten-day stay in the hospital, Alison's mother never left Alison's sight. She was there when Alison started to hallucinate because of all the medications she had been given; when Alison was running a high fever after the surgery; and when some of the many IVs in Alison's body (put there because Alison preferred IVs to shots) kept slipping out of her veins. Though the first couple of days after Alison's surgery were difficult to endure, Alison got through them with the help of her mother.

After those first few post-operative days, Alison started to feel like herself again. She was socially outgoing in the pediatric ward of the hospital, received many visitors, and entertained everyone in the hospital. Her ceaseless energy and rambunctious nature could not be quelled—not even by a scoliosis surgery.

Surgery #2: Before Sophomore Year: Toward the end of freshman year, Alison began to feel better and went back to cheerleading. Almost a year had passed since her spine fusion, and she was ready to get back to her normal activities. That summer, when Alison visited her orthopedic doctor for a checkup, she was surprised to see on her X rays that part of the instrumentation in her spine had "popped loose." Alison's mother attributed the dissemblance of the rod system to Alison's having taken part in the last few cheerleading practices of the year. Regardless of *why* Alison's Harrington rod had come undone, the fact was that it had come undone and had to be removed. At the age of fifteen, during the summer before her sophomore year in high school, Alison underwent her second scoliosis-related surgery and had her rod removed.

The rod removal surgery was relatively simple in comparison to the major spine fusion Alison had undergone the summer before. When they removed the rods, the doctors saw that Alison's spine had fused in its straight position anyway, so the presence of the rods in her back was no longer necessary. Alison was up and out of the hospital in just a few days after this second surgery, and she was able to go back to cheerleading during her sophomore year.

Surgery #3: Before Junior Year: One day during the summer before her junior year in high school, Alison was moving furniture. All of a sudden she felt something in her back "pop"—she did not know at the time that her fusion had broken. Alison's actual spine was still in one piece, but the overlying layer of bone—the fusion made of bone graft—had broken. With no rods and no fusion to hold it in place, Alison's spine would continue to curve just as it had prior to any of the surgeries. In order for Alison's scoliosis to be corrected—even to be stopped at this point—she would have to have another spinal fusion. When Alison's doctor recommended surgery, Alison said, "No way." She had already endured two surgeries and was absolutely not going to endure a third. Then her doctor said something that changed her mind immediately.

"My doctor scared me to death by telling me that I could be paralyzed before the age of twenty-one if I did not have this surgery," Alison says. With that having been said, Alison and her family decided that surgery was in order. At age sixteen, Alison had her third surgery. Her doctor inserted more rods and put more bone graft atop the rods to fuse Alison's spine in a straight position once and for all.

Following this surgery, Alison found herself feeling particularly uncomfortable—perhaps because the doctor had to break the rest of Alison's old fusion before he inserted the rods and made a new fusion, or perhaps because Alison's body was just getting tired of all this surgery. She felt more pain now than she had after the previous two surgeries. Alison did have homebound tutoring for the first few weeks of her junior year in school. She was so intrinsically energetic, though, that she craved some sort of activity. So, while she had trouble sitting in a chair, Alison began dancing again at Ballet Florida. She was in a post-operative body cast at the time, so she had to forego a lot of the exercises done in ballet class. But she felt better being up, out, and exercising than she had felt at home in bed. The culmination of Alison's junior year—like the culmination of most junior years—ended in her taking the SAT's. While most people worry about wearing layered clothing and drinking water to maintain their comfort during the test, Alison showed up at the testing site in her body cast, ready to do her best despite her uncomfortable situation.

Surgery #4: Before Senior Year: Alison was seventeen in 1985 when she traveled to Germany with her class during the summer before she began her senior year. One dark, rainy night, the group of high school kids and chaperones was touring a variety of locations in Germany. At one point, Alison was running down a flight of stairs to catch the tour bus before it departed for its next location, and she happened to trip and fall. As soon as she felt trails of excruciating pain running up and down her spine, she knew that her rods had broken.

Alison's teachers escorted her to the bus and watched while she sat there screaming in pain. The tour bus then drove to three different hospitals trying to get help. At one hospital, a doctor had taken X rays of Alison and, upon seeing the X rays, Alison knew that she had been right; the rod was broken. Alison's German teacher would try to interpret to doctors what Alison—who was now as familiar with scoliosis as the doctors were—said was wrong with her. At 2:00 A.M., after four hours of jumping from hospital to hospital, one hospital agreed to take Alison and operate on her.

In response to the hospital's offer, Alison simply said, "No, I'll miss my plane if I stay here." She asked the doctor at the hospital to give her some pain pills and told her teachers that she would take the next available flight to America. Everyone did as Alison told them, and the next day Alison returned home. Her frantic parents met her at the airport and drove her straight from the airport to the hospital where, in an emergency surgery, Alison's rods were removed. Luckily, Alison's fusion had already taken place. Her spine was straight, and it was fixed solidly into position.

After a high school experience complete with four consecutive sco-liosis surgeries, earning the nickname "Turtle," and four "coming-out-of-cast" parties, Alison graduated in the spring of 1986. She received a scholarship to the University of Tampa and worked at a horseback rid-ing stable in addition to attending college. Alison continued to take dance classes throughout college and also learned how to foxhunt.

In 1989, at the age of twenty-one, Alison got married. Three years later, she gave birth to her son Kyle, whom she calls "the joy of [her] life." During her pregnancy, Alison did not experience any back-related problems. Interestingly, she had not been aware of the fact that her having had a spine fusion had made her unable to have an epidural. So, in the absence of an epidural, Alison had a normal birth via "seventeen hours of hard labor, determination, and a wonderful husband." Her baby was a normal, healthy, seven-pound, six-ounce boy with no prob-lems whatsoever.

Presently, Alison's dream is to start a horse program for children with emotional difficulties. Considering the determination, energy, and initiative she has shown throughout her life, I have no doubt that Alison will fulfill this dream very soon.

SONDRA

"A sense of gratitude is the greatest gift you can give yourself."

I arrived at a penthouse apartment in Palm Beach and knocked on the door not knowing what to expect. The woman who answered my knock was a beautiful blonde who immediately impressed me with her evident poise and elegance.

"Come in," she said, smiling a magnetic smile. She held the door open as I walked in, and as I passed by her I caught a whiff of her light, sweet-smelling perfume. From the opposite side of the apartment, a warm breeze passed through an open glass door that led to a terrace peering out at the sparkling blue Atlantic. Rays of sun shone through the open terrace door and illuminated the multitude of paintings that covered the walls of the apartment.

"You must like art," I said to the woman.

"Yes," she answered. "I painted all of the paintings you see on my walls."

At first, I did not believe her. But as I began talking to Sondra and came to know her, I fully believed that she had painted every one of the paintings that decorated her apartment. A piece of paper displaying quotations from reviews of Sondra's artwork ultimately convinced me that the professional-looking paintings I saw had been done by Sondra—the widowed artist and scoliosis patient whom I was presently talking to:

> Sondra's unique and individual creations unfold from a boundless imagination. They are vibrant with color, romantic in quality, and rich in texture. The technique she uses is reminiscent of the great French Impressionists.
> —Alexander Sideris

> Her paintings have a significant place in our troubled world today... they express love and gentleness.
> —The Daily Palm Beacher

> The ethereal quality of Sondra's paointings project her thoughtful fantasies, pleasing both the mind and the heart.
> —Palm Beach Illustrated

Throughout her life, Sondra has been thoughtful, imaginative, and creative. Sondra's creativity is unique in that it did not emerge on its own but, rather, out of necessity. At the age of fourteen, she found herself trapped in a plaster body cast that extended from under her arms to her hips and reached down her right leg. For five months, Sondra lay flat on her back and unable to move in a bed in her unairconditioned home. She used knitting needles to scratch her itches. She went to the bathroom in a bedpan. And she waited patiently while her mother turned her body sideways in the bed, sat in a chair next to her, put her hair in a basin, and washed her hair. In addition to withstanding the troubles of everyday living in a body cast, Sondra went through puberty in that cast. She got her first period while she was in the cast and had to lay in bed, motionless, enduring terrible menstrual cramps.

It was while she was in her body cast that Sondra developed her creativity. The only way she was able to cope with the agony of having to lay trapped and motionless for five months was to free her mind; the only way she could transcend the pain of having to wear a rough, heavy

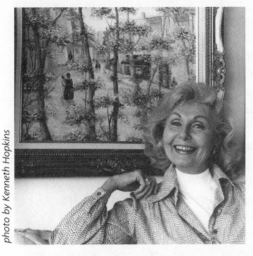

photo by Kenneth Hopkins

body cast was to imagine that she was elsewhere.

"Mentally, I used to walk in my mind," Sondra remembers. "I would take [imaginary] walks in my mind, out the door and down the stairs, out the front door and around the corner, up over the hill and then I'd come back." The imaginative creativity Sondra was forced to develop as a fourteen-year-old trapped in a body cast has stayed with her throughout her life.

The jailor that placed Sondra in that body cast was scoliosis. She had been diagnosed in 1946 by her physical education teacher. Her teacher had noticed that Sondra had remarkably poor posture and had suggested that Sondra's mother take Sondra to a doctor. Soon afterward, Sondra had found herself in the office of an orthopedic doctor who said that she did have scoliosis but that she should wait to see how the scoliosis would behave and return to his office in six months. When Sondra returned to the orthopedic surgeon six months later, the surgeon recommended surgery.

"Nobody had even heard of scoliosis surgery in 1946," Sondra says. "I was told that I would be crippled with serious complications if I didn't have the surgery, so I ended up having it."

Just six months after her physical education teacher had noticed her poor posture, Sondra was fused from her T6 vertebra to her L5 vertebra. No rods were used in the surgery; in 1946, the technique was used just to straighten the spine, put bone graft on it, and hope it fused in that straight position. It was for this reason that the body cast was necessary. Without instrumentation to hold it in place, the fusing spine might have sunk back into its curved position post-operatively. To prevent this, Sondra was placed in a full body cast for more than five months after her surgery. The part of the cast that extended down her right leg was crafted by the doctor to ensure that Sondra would not be able to move during her months of recovery.

"It [the cast] went all the way around my whole body and down my leg to my knee so that I could not move," Sondra says. "They did not want me to move."

Sondra was semiconscious for three days immediately following the surgery. She remembers being only vaguely aware of anything during those days because the hospital staff kept her "pretty sedated." Sondra was in the hospital for one month following the surgery; then she was discharged to go home and recover.

Before the torso of her body cast was ever sawed off, the leg portion was removed. Sondra remembers being in bed at her home and seeing her leg all "atrophied and scaly" from having been in a cast for so long. When she attempted to stand up, she collapsed. It took Sondra weeks after that to gain the strength back in her right leg and to learn how to walk while wearing a fifty-pound cast.

Throughout her trying months of recovery from her scoliosis surgery, Sondra found the strength to persevere and to focus on the future in the creative visions her mind conjured. When she wasn't going on mental walks and saving herself from the dementia that inevitably awaits anyone who has been isolated for so long, Sondra was praying to God.

"I was not a religious person at all," she admits. "But I believed in God. Somehow I always felt that God was my friend. I felt that he was watching over me, and that was very comforting to me. I remember I wasn't angry about having the operation. I was more curious because I always thought bad things happened to bad people. I didn't think bad things happened to good people, and I thought I was a good person. I was very curious at fourteen as to why this had happened to me. I asked God why this had happened to me. The answer that I got was that I could never take anything for granted."

Even today, fifty-three years after she had her surgery, Sondra does not take anything for granted. She appreciates every walk and continues to view even a simple bath as a luxury. Her time spent in pain and in a body cast gave Sondra an appreciation for life and its small pleasures that have lasted her a lifetime.

Sondra now has strong feelings about the importance of maintaining body condition, mental health, and scoliosis pain control by way of "any exercise regime that works for you." Frequent exercise has helped Sondra deal with her pain for the past forty years and has made her a firm believer in its power to heal.

In addition to exercise, Sondra recommends meditation, biofeedback, finding or making (audio) tapes that administer music therapy, and developing a hobby to help transcend pain as treatments for those scoliosis patients who are not surgical candidates. Sondra's therapeutic hobby of choice happens to be art. This hobby of imagining—which originated in Sondra's mind when she was fourteen and in a body cast— has now materialized into a collection of beautiful paintings and has become her life's work.

In addition to painting, Sondra enjoys writing and feels that writing is a very important exercise for people dealing with physical problems. She recommends keeping a journal for anyone who *has* constant physical complaints. Writing—instead of complaining constantly to people—is, according to Sondra, a very healthy thing to do.

"I let people know that I'm not just a pretty blonde standing here with no problems," she says. "I tell them my story so that they realize that we're overcoming all the time in life. A sense of gratitude is the greatest gift you can give yourself."

Sondra's curves have now progressed to thirty-seven degrees in the thoracic region and sixty-four degrees in the lumbar region. None of the doctors she has seen about her scoliosis sees a need to operate. Sondra has obtained a support brace similar to a small corset, though, which she always wears for comfort.

"I have a maid who comes in once a week to change the linens on the beds, because I can't lift the mattresses," Sondra says, admitting to her scoliosis-related limitations. "I really don't lift anything heavy. But I can bend. I can exercise. And I'm very good in bed! When my husband used to take me around to the doctors, I used to say, 'If I could walk around with a mattress, I would have no troubles!' "

When Sondra said this to me during our conversation, my mouth dropped open. I laughed at her sudden outpouring of candid eccentricity and said, "You're so funny!"

"I have to have a sense of humor," she responded, smiling. "I have to laugh because if you don't laugh, you cry. If you cry, it's bad for the face. Got to keep laughing—it's the best medicine."

Chapter 5

Indications for Surgery

Skeletal maturity, curve flexibility, curve magnitude, success with bracing or other nonoperative treatments, physical appearance, pulmonary function, and general health are the factors doctors consider when they determine whether you are a candidate for surgery. Your *skeletal maturity* indicates how much growth you have remaining; the more growth you have left, the more your scoliosis curve will progress. And the more severe your curve is once you have reached skeletal maturity, the greater your risk is of experiencing progression into adulthood. Your *curve flexibility* indicates how far your spine is capable of being straightened; the more flexible your curve, the greater scoliosis correction your doctor can achieve in surgery. Having and maintaining a flexible curve with a mild to moderate change in curve magnitude may also enable you to postpone surgery for a few years and to still attain a similar degree of correction when you *do* decide to have surgery, as you would if you had undergone surgery sooner. Your *curve magnitude* simply indicates how severe your scoliosis is and serves as an objective standard by which your doctor can judge your need for surgery. The success you have had with *bracing or other nonoperative treatments* indicates how easily your curvature can be controlled or detained. If bracing was successful for you, you may not need to have surgery; if bracing was unsuccessful for you, your only remaining treatment option is surgery. *Physical appearance* is usually more important to the patient than it is to the doctor. If you express a lot of concern about uneven hips or a prominent rib hump, your doctor may recommend surgery to improve your cosmetic appearance. If, however, you are not bothered by your deformity and there are not other indications to have surgery, then your doctor will not be as likely to recommend that you have surgery. *Pulmonary function* indicates the effect of curvature and spinal rotation on your breathing. A severely curved and rotated spine will ultimately cause a compression of the internal organs—including the lungs—and will slowly decrease your breathing capacity. If this is the case, your scoliosis has progressed to a potentially dangerous level, making it more likely that your doctor will recommend surgery. If you are in *good health*, your surgery should run smoothly and you should be resilient enough to recover quickly. If you are in *poor health*, however, doctors may hesitate to recommend surgery to you; if you are experiencing health problems more serious than scoliosis, doctors will likely encourage you to treat your other problems before treating your scoliosis. And if your poor health is a result of your scoliosis, doctors are likely to recommend surgery at the earliest possible convenience to correct your curvature and improve your overall well-being.

There are two groups of patients who fall into the broad category of "surgical candidates." The first group comprises adolescents whose scoliosis is equal to or exceeds fifty degrees in measurement. Studies prove that curves measuring fifty degrees cannot be treated effectively by any means other than surgery. The second group comprises people with progressive scoliosis curves who have reached skeletal maturity. Once you have reached skeletal maturity, bracing and other nonoperative treatments are ineffective means of treating your scoliosis. The only treatment that can improve or correct a scoliosis curve in a mature patient is surgery. Nonprogressive adults with curves who are experiencing pain are also considered surgical candidates.

Though each scoliosis case is unique, and doctors choose to perform or not to perform surgery for various, legitimate reasons that arise in the cases with which they are presented, the aforementioned indicators can be trusted to determine, in general, which patients are surgical candidates and which are not. The goals of surgery are to arrest the progressive deformity associated with worsening scoliosis and to produce a painless, stable, balanced spine held by a solid fusion. If achieving any of these goals would improve your health, your self-confidence, and/or your lifestyle, assume it is an indication that surgery may be the right choice for you.

PRE-OPERATIVE ACTIVITY

Once you and your doctor have decided that surgery is an appropriate treatment for your scoliosis, you need to mentally and physically prepare yourself for your surgery.

MENTAL PREPARATION

Before you have surgery, it is important that you become as comfortable as possible with the hospital, surgical protocol, and the idea of having surgery. If knowing absolutely nothing about the surgery or the hospital puts you at ease, or if remaining unaware of exactly what will happen to you during the surgery makes you most comfortable, do not hesitate to inform your parents, spouse, friends, or doctor of that. If, on the other hand, knowing everything about the hospital and the surgical method that will be applied to you makes you feel most comfortable, feel free to ask your doctor any questions you may have.

If you are the type of person who wishes to know exactly what will go on in the course of your imminent surgery and recovery, you may also ask your doctor for videos and an information packet concerning scoliosis surgery (most doctors will have these readily available). Certain hospitals—especially children's hospitals—even offer patients the opportunity to visit the hospital for a day before having surgery. On such a day, you will be led through the steps you will have to follow when you return to actually have surgery; in other words, a day spent visiting the hospital is often a good "practice run" for you to take before plunging into "the real thing." If, during a visit to the hospital, you do not understand something, ask a doctor or nurse to explain it to you. Even in the days and hours before your actual surgery, feel free to ask the doctors and nurses what they are doing to you or where they are taking you. After all, if knowing what is going on makes you feel more comfortable, then do not hesitate to find out what is going on!

PHYSICAL PREPARATION

Not only do you need to prepare your mind and your spirit for your surgery, but you need to prepare your body as well. Feeling healthy and energetic and being in shape right before you have surgery can only help you. Good health can actually make your time spent in the hospital faster, less painful, and easier to endure; it can also expedite your total recovery period by enabling you to sit, stand, walk, and function more easily after surgery. Be sure to ask your doctor for his or her suggestions concerning presurgical nutrition, muscle exercises, and breathing exercises. And try to be mindful of your health and attentive to your doctor's suggestions in the weeks or months leading up to your surgery. After your surgery, you will reap the rewards of your efforts.

SOME QUESTIONS YOU MAY WANT TO ASK YOUR DOCTOR

- What amount of correction can we expect?
- Will the thoracic lordosis be corrected?
- Will the lumbar rotation be corrected?
- What is the length of the operation?
- What is the amount of blood loss expected?
- How much blood should be donated beforehand?
- What approach will be used—anterior? posterior? a combination? Why? If a combination, will the surgery be on one day or in stages?
- What is the protocol for communication between the operating room and the patient's family during surgery? (It is a long operation, and the waiting is stressful.)
- What is the doctor's schedule in the weeks following surgery? Will he/she be around in the event of a complication?
- What are the policies of the hospital (for intensive care, special care, the pediatric ward, the adult unit) allowing a parent to stay overnight with a patient?
- Does the hospital offer tours?
- Can the surgery be performed endoscopically—using a thoracoscope—through the portholes?
- Will the rods used be pediatric size? If not, then what size are they?
- Will the type of hooks used be low-profile?
- What type of instrumentation will be used? (There have been

newer designs in rods and modifications that have been made since their introduction; also, if they are stainless steel or titanium, consider a metal allergy, though this is very rare.)

- Does the doctor use steri-strips over the incision?
- What can be expected in the recuperation period—starting with immediate post-op to full recovery?
- What limitations are there post-operatively, from initial post-op to full recovery. (For example, bending is quite limited at the initial phases but increases with time.)
- How much physical therapy is needed post-operatively? Is it usual to need physical therapy once home from the hospital?
- Will any kind of bracing be needed after the surgery?
- Are there medical aids that will be needed during the recuperation? (For example, a toilet seat extender or a gripper; if yes, does the hospital or a medical supply store supply these?)
- How long will the hospital stay be?
- How soon will you be sitting? standing? walking? eating? climbing stairs?
- What is the timetable for the removal of the IV's, monitors, catheter tube, etc.?
- Can the doctor explain the hospital consent form?

You can also:

- Ask for extra time to be allotted to your doctor's appointments so you can ask all of your questionsin a relaxed, nonrushed space.
- Ask your doctor to give explanations for his/her decisions. (This is a good general rule to go by.)
- Ask the doctor for names of other patients to whom he/she could refer you.
- Ask for an M.D. anesthesiologist and not a certified nurse anesthesiologist.
- Ask for a timetable to resume activities—perhaps broken down into one week, one month, three months, six months, and one year. Include things such as bicycling, light jogging, routine gym classes, noncontact sports, horseback riding—no jumping, skiing—water and snow, gymnastics, parachuting, dirt bike racing, roller coasters and amusement park rides, contact sports, lifting more than ten pounds, skateboarding, surfing, bungee jumping, motorcycling, etc.

PREPARATION FOR SURGERY

Before having surgery, you will need to sign a consent form, similar to the example below. Before presenting you with the consent form, your doctor will have a discussion with you about the section of the form that reads, "The nature . . . and consequences of such a . . . procedure . . . have been explained and discussed with me by [my doctor]." The potential "consequences" of surgery that your doctor will warn you about are a series of complications including paralysis and even death. *Do not worry* when you hear these words. Though events such as paralysis and death have occurred in past surgeries, the incidence of such complications is *extremely* low.[23] Your doctor is obliged to discuss with you all the *possible* complications that may occur during surery because of legal reasons.

CONSENT FORM FOR OPERATION and/or PROCEDURE

I hereby give consent to Dr. _____ and associates or assistants of his/her choice and the _____ Hospital and its staff to provide such surgical procedures and therapeutic services as they consider necessary, including the following operation and/or procedure described as:

_____

_____

(describe operation and/or procedure)

upon_____.

(name of patient)

The nature, purpose, benefits, foreseeable risks, complications and consequences of such an operation/procedure, as well as the alternatives to the above operation/procedure, have been explained and discussed with me by _____.

(name of physician)

I give this permission with full knowledge and understanding thereof. I understand that medicine is not an exact science and that there exists a possibility that the operation/procedure may not have the results intended. I am also aware that there are always risks and dangers to life and health associated with surgery, use of medication, medical procedures and treatments which can cause adverse consequences not usually anticipated in advance, but I give this permission with full assent nevertheless.

I understand that during the course of the operation/procedure, unforeseen conditions may arise that necessitate surgical or other additional procedures different from those contemplated. I therefore authorize the above named physician or his/her designees to perform such additional surgical or other procedures as are deemed necessary.

I have read and fully understand the above and have been given the opportunity to ask questions, and all my questions have been answered adequately.

I represent to my/the patient's physician and the _____ Hospital that I am eligible to give this consent.*

Signature of patient/parent/guardian _____

Date _____

Relationship to patient _____

*If the patient is under 18 years of age, the patient's parent or legal guardian must give permission, unless the patient has married or is the parent of a child.

In addition to signing a consent form prior to your surgery, you must undergo a series of routine tests and blood donations. These noninvasive tests include a pulmonary function test and a neurological examination. The purpose of these tests is to make certain that your breathing capacity, brain function, and central nervous system function are normal and to provide a basis for comparison of your breathing capacity, brain function, and central nervous system function after surgery.

The blood donations that are requested of you prior to your having surgery serve the purpose of forming an autologous blood bank that will be drawn from during your surgery. It is likely that your doctor will ask you to come to the hospital a couple of times before your surgery (perhaps one month before and then two weeks before) to donate your own blood. This blood will then be transfused into you in the operating room to replace the blood you lose during your surgery. Donating your own blood prior to having surgery prevents you from having to use blood from a blood bank—which happens to be carefully screened and very safe to use, anyway—and absolutely ensures that the blood used during your surgery is clean, pure, and untainted. If you are anemic or are uneasy about the idea of having to give blood prior to surgery, ask family members or close friends whose blood types are the same as or compatible with yours to donate blood for you. This sort of arrangement is not uncommon.

SURGICAL METHODS

The goals of surgery are to obtain balance, correction of the scoliosis, a solid fusion, preservation of as many motion segments as possible, and as near anatomic alignment as possible. There are two means of attaining these goals. The first is simply implants into the spine. The second is supplementing the implants with a fusion of the bones and joints in the spine. Spine instrumentation entails the attachment of a system of metal devices (hooks, wires, screws, rods, etc.) to the spine. This system of metal implants will vary in length according to the magnitude and location of the curve. The hooks, screws, and wires are essentially anchored into the vertebrae, and the rods are placed in the anchors for fixation. The rods are then cranked or rotated to straighten the spine. A fusion of the spine entails the spreading of bone graft over the joints and vertebrae, which have already been straightened by the metal implants. As the bone graft ossifies, it fuses with the spine; this newly formed fusion of bone graft and vertebrae ensures that the spine will permanently be held in its new, corrected position.

Insertion of implants without a

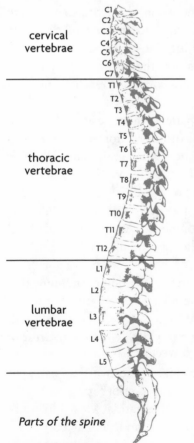

cervical vertebrae

C1
C2
C3
C4
C5
C6
C7

thoracic vertebrae

T1
T2
T3
T4
T5
T6
T7
T8
T9
T10
T11
T12

lumbar vertebrae

L1
L2
L3
L4
L5

Parts of the spine

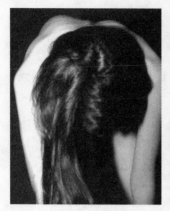 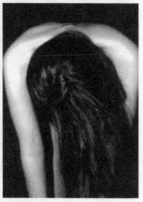

Left: Preoperative forward bend. Note the rotational prominence (hump).

Right: Postoperative forward bend. Note the correction of the thoracic hump.

fusion—achieved by using the subcutaneous rod program[24]—is recommended for very young patients who are not through growing. Fusing the spine of a patient who is still growing would thwart further growth of the spine, thereby creating a short trunk as the rest of the body grows. Still, curves that are corrected using just subcutaneous rods will eventually need to be reinforced by a fusion; the fusion surgery is usually performed once patients with subcutaneous rods reach prepuberty age (before adolescent growth spurt).

The mainstay of scoliosis surgery for patients (teenage and adult) who have reached skeletal maturity is spinal fusion reinforced by implants. Such a fusion is obtained by the placement of bone graft material, either obtained from the rib or from the iliac crest (pelvic bone), onto the spinal segments and joints. Though the bone graft is placed in, on, and around the vertebrae during surgery, it does not actually fuse until several months after the surgery has been completed. As a general rule, doctors say that the entire fusion process takes approximately six months to one year. This is why doctors will tell you not to return to your "normal" level of physical activity (not to return to doing anything that might harm your impressionable, fusing spine) for an entire year following your surgery. Once the fusion of bone has been achieved, your spine is solid and strong enough to remain straightened for the rest of your life.

There are a variety of surgical approaches used to treat scoliosis. The most widely accepted surgical approach is the posterior (approaching the spine from the back) spinal fusion with instrumentation. Most adolescent and young adult thoracic and double thoracic and lumbar curves are treated in this fashion. Historically, the surgical instrumentation and

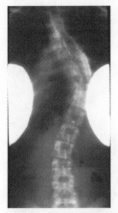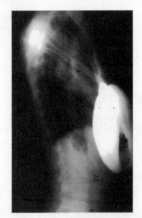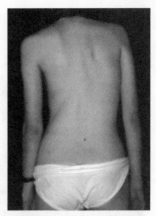

Above: Preoperative spinal X rays from the back and side and preoperative photo

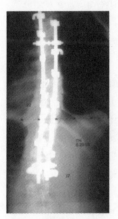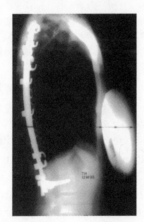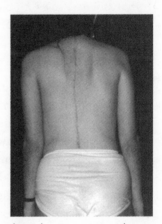

Above: Postoperative spinal X rays from the back and side and postoperative photo

practice of posterior fusion began with the Harrington rod system, which achieved correction of the lateral curvature associated with scoliosis by means of a simple distraction and compression of the vertebrae. More recently, other instrumentation and implant systems have superannuated Harrington rods and have come to correct both the lateral curvature and the rotation associated with scoliosis. These multisegmental hook, screw, and wire fixation systems provide multiple forms of scoliosis correction, as they allow for distraction, compression, rotation, and translation of the vertebrae all at once. The more modern fixation systems also allow maintenance of the normal sagittal (side) contours of kyphosis and lordosis that the Harrington rod system did not maintain. In other words,

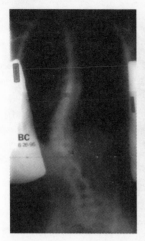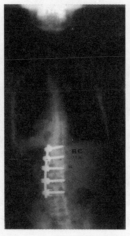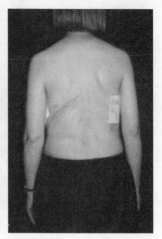

*Forty-year-old female with lumbar scoliosis treated with selective anterior fusion and instrumentation. **Left:** Preoperative X ray. **Center:** Postoperative X ray. **Right:** Postoperative photo. Note the incision on the patient's side.*

modern instrumentation and implant systems allow you to maintain normal amounts of roundback and swayback, whereas Harrington rod systems tended to make your entire spine abnormally flat in the side plane, especially in the implant was extended to the lower lumbar spine. In addition, these new instrumentation systems eliminate the need for the postoperative body casts and braces that were used in conjunction with Harrington rod and in the days prior to spinal instrumentation. Studies show that the curve correction achieved with any of the following instrumentation systems is fifty to eighty percent. Each of the following systems has nuances that set it apart from the rest. Doctors choose which instrumentation systems to use in given situations, based on the nature of the patient's scoliosis and on their own preferences for particular systems.

The Different Instrumentation and Implant Systems
Harrington
Cotrel-Dubousset
Isola
Luque
Moss Miami
Synergy
TSRH (Texas Scottish Rite Hospital)

TITANIUM VS. STAINLESS STEEL

Titanium systems made their appearance on the market about two years ago. Since that time, I have met many people who have had titanium instrumentation (see Anthony, page 221, and Zoe, page 224). This raises the obvious question about the differences between stainless steel and titanium—a question I am frequently asked.

Since titanium use is relatively new there are, to date, no conclusive studies done regarding the behavior of this material. What we do know, however, are the advantages and disadvantages. The advantages of titanium include:

- it is light weight;
- it doesn't cause an allergic reaction—patients with strong allergies to nickel, which is found in stainless steel, do best with titanium, which has a very low allergy potential (see Sherry, page 232);
- there is better post-operative imaging with an MRI or a CAT scan (which is not possible with stainless steel);
- may be more flexible (though less resistant to breakage);
- if a patient has pain later in life, it is more visible.

The disadvantages of titanium include:

- it is more expensive;
- it is more difficult to use, especially for complex curves;
- may not be as strong as stainless steel;
- it has a tendency to break if nicks occur within portions of the implant.

Discuss these differences with your doctor and ask which system he/she plans to use so that you will know in the future. Your doctor is the one best equipped to make this decision.

THE ROLE OF ANTERIOR SURGERY

Anterior (approaching the spine from the front) approaches to scoliosis surgery have recently become more common. In comparison with posterior surgery, anterior surgery is a more involved operation because it involves temporarily shifting some internal organs in order to reach the spine from the front. And, while posterior surgery results in a vertical scar straight down the back, anterior surgery results in a slanting scar on one side of the chest or abdomen (along or right below the rib cage).

The anterior approach to scoliosis surgery is known for "obtaining correction, insuring fusions, and allowing better alignment of the scoliotic spine over fewer segments."[25] Yet anterior surgery is only recommended for a select group of scoliosis cases; the anterior procedure is generally used to treat thoracolumbar and lumbar scoliosis. Recently, the anterior approach is also being extended to treat thoracic curves, which traditionally have been treated from a posterior approach. The reports regarding such treatments are too early to judge the actual advantages and disadvantages of approaching the thoracic spine anteriorly.

The advantages of treating thoracolumbar and lumbar curves with an anterior approach is to fuse a shorter segment of the spine, thereby freeing up motion segments above and below the fusion. In other words, an anterior approach to surgery will allow the patient to maintain a greater range of motion in the spine than would a posterior approach. Anterior surgery also provides anterior growth arrest of the spine and, therefore, prevents the crankshaft phenomenon[26] that occurs in skeletally immature patients who are treated with posterior surgery alone.

If maintaining the range of motion in your spine is a matter of great importance to you, ask doctors about the possibility of approaching your scoliosis anteriorly. Know, though, that anterior surgery is not a substitute for posterior surgery. If doctors you consult seem to feel that your particular curve can be better treated by a posterior approach to surgery, do not persist about wanting to have anterior surgery instead. Some approaches are right for some curves; other approaches are right for other curves.

COMBINED ANTERIOR AND POSTERIOR SURGERY

If you have a very severe thoracic, thoracolumbar, or lumbar scoliosis curve, you may be a candidate for a combined anterior and poste-

rior approach to surgery. This is the most complex of scoliosis surgeries because it involves approaching the spine from both the front
and the back. The first step in this surgery is the anterior release,
which entails anterior disc removal. The spine is approached anteriorly and is fused without instrumentation in order to release the spine
and to provide flexibility to the vertebral column. This step is followed by the second step, which is the posterior approach. The posterior portion of this surgery usually occurs either under the same
anesthetic or a few days to a week after the anterior surgery. The posterior portion of the surgery involves a spinal fusion *with* instrumentation. Recent studies have shown that patients treated with
combined procedures under the same anesthetic on the same day fare
better than those treated a few days to a week apart. Having both the
anterior and the posterior portions of this surgery on the same day
results in fewer complications from wound healing, nutritional problems, and anesthetic administration—and results in a shorter hospital
stay.

THE THORACOSCOPIC APPROACH TO SURGERY

The newest approach to scoliosis surgery is the thoracoscopic
approach. This involves approaching the spine from a series of small
porthole incisions on the side of the body as opposed to larger incisions in the front or back of the body. There is a scope (a little camera)
on the tip of the instrument used to do this surgery. The scope is inserted through these small (inch-long) incisions and produces an image of
the spine on a television screen in the operating room. Since the spine
is not exposed in this type of surgery, the doctor views it and performs
the removal of disc and the fusion of it by looking at the television
screen.

The main advantage of a thoracoscopic approach to surgery is that it
is minimally invasive. Instead of having any large, visible scars after
surgery, you will have a few very small scars. However, this technique
can only be used to fuse the spine anteriorly at this point. And,
although it has been generally successful in the instances in which it has
been used to fuse the spine, the thoracoscopic spinal instrumentation
surgery is not widely practiced as the standard of care. It is still viewed
as being relatively new and as needing to prove its consistency and legit-

imacy. General applications of this new technique still require documentation and clinical reports.

THORACOPLASTY

A thoracoplasty is not another approach to surgery; it is not even a means of correcting scoliosis. A thoracoplasty is a procedure sometimes performed in conjunction with a spine fusion. It involves the removal of rib segments associated with thoracic scoliosis patients.

Scoliosis-related rotation of the spine often results in a visible rotation of the rib cage. This rotation of the rib cage is the origin of any "hump" (presumably a *rib* hump) you may see as a manifestation of your deformity. The rib prominence can be improved by a thoracoplasty. Once your doctor has placed the instrumentation in your spine during surgery, he or she can move on to your ribs and remove portions of the more protruding ribs. This removal of rib segments decreases your "hump" and greatly improves your cosmetic appearance. It may also provide your doctor with enough bone from which to make bone graft so that he or she does not have to take any bone from your iliac crest—the place from which material for bone graft is usually taken.

If you are considering a thoracoplasty, you need not worry about having a lack of rib segments once the procedure has been completed. Ribs grow back when they are cut, yet the new parts of the ribs tend to be softer, less rigid, and less prominent. Also, a mild (ten to fifteen percent) decrease in pulmonary function can be an aftereffect of a thoracoplasty, but full pulmonary function usually returns in just one to two years.

IN THE OPERATING ROOM

The operating room contains more people and machines during surgery than you might expect. While your doctor and his or her team of assisting doctors and residents concern themselves with the surgery, other people in the operating room concern themselves with your brain, your spinal cord, your nerves, your anesthesia, your vital signs, and your general well-being.

Nurses are in charge of inserting your catheter tubes and assisting the anesthesiologist. They also make sure that your blood is flowing through your body and limbs during the surgery and that you are receiving blood transfusions to replace the blood you lose during the surgery. An anesthesiologist sits beside a machine that indicates your vital signs, administers your anesthesia, maintains a safe drug level in your body, and is ready to alert the doctor if anything goes wrong. Similarly, a neurologist or monitoring neurotechnologist sits beside a machine—a kind of neurological monitor—which indicates your brain and spinal cord function and the safety of your spinal cord during the procedure. If the instrumentation comes close to your spinal cord during the surgery, the monitor will indicate it, and the technologist or neurologist will alert the doctor so that spinal cord damage can be prevented—the most critical phase is during the correction of the curve.

In addition to the neurologic and anesthetic types of monitors that are in the operating room during surgery, there are other apparatuses present to ensure your safety and well-being. Compression boots with Velcro wraps (much like the ones used when your physician is checking your blood pressure) are placed around your limbs; they periodically tighten and then loosen again in order to keep your blood circulating. A machine called a cell saver is present during the surgery as well. The cell saver extracts the blood from the operative wound. It cleans and processes the blood, then transfuses it back into your body. In essence, the cell saver recycles your lost blood and slightly lessens the need for the transfusion of other, stored blood into your body.

IMMEDIATELY FOLLOWING SURGERY

Immediately after your surgery, you are transferred from the operating room to the post-anesthesia recovery room or intensive care unit. Most people remain in these units for at least twenty-four hours (if not more) before being moved into a regular hospital recovery room. When you wake up, you will probably have some IVs and tubes still attached to you. These are present to hydrate you, to nourish you, to lessen your pain, and to take care of your excretory needs (you will not be able to get up and go to the bathroom for, perhaps, one or two days). If these IVs and tubes bother you, do not worry; they will be removed in just a matter of days.

Once you demonstrate signs of being relatively stable and well, the hospital personnel will bring you to have post-operative X rays taken. Some patients describe this process as being the most painful aspect of their entire hospital experience; other patients disagree. The post-operative X rays may be painful for you because you have *just* come out of surgery and you are now being transferred to different areas of the hospital and moved around on an uncomfortable X-ray table. This process happens quickly, though, and soon you are back in your hospital bed. These X rays are now often done in the operating room while the patient is still under anesthesia. The post-operative X rays will indicate the degree of scoliosis correction that was attained during surgery. Do not expect your spine to be completely straight after surgery; that is seldom the case. But *do* expect to see that you have achieved a considerable degree of scoliosis correction by having surgery, and remember that the correction surgery achieves always varies with patients' curve magnitude and curve flexibility.

Doctors and nurses will check on you periodically throughout your stay in the hospital. Still, if at all possible, you should have a parent, spouse, or good friend stay with you at all times. Having someone who cares about you by your side ensures that everything is being done to benefit you and to hasten your recovery. A parent, spouse, or good friend may bring you added comfort or may notice something that your doctors and nurses do not and can bring this to the doctors' and nurses' attentions.

For pain management immediately after surgery, you will most likely have a supply of morphine to administer by yourself. Your doctors and nurses will set the morphine at a level they feel is appropriate; there is a limit put on how much morphine you can access because your doctors and nurses do not want you to accidentally overdose on the pain-killing drug. Whenever you feel pain, you may push a button, and you will receive a dosage of morphine from your ready supply. The button will lock once you have reached your limit.

The speed of recovery varies from person to person. Being healthy and fit before surgery, keeping yourself well-hydrated throughout your hospital stay, and *wanting* to get better should facilitate the quickest, easiest recovery possible.

POST-OPERATIVE ACTIVITIES

"Statistically, significant improvements [have been] seen in post-operative scores for physical function, social function, bodily pain, and perceived health change."[27] In most cases, people who have had surgery

look and feel notably better than they did prior to surgery. This looking and feeling better, however, may not arrive immediately after your
surgery. For the first few days, weeks, or even months following your
surgery, you may not feel quite like yourself. It will take some time
before you stop feeling pain and fatigue and start feeling pain-free and
energetic again. It will also take some time to redevelop your appetite,
your desire to go out, and your interest in various activities. It is important to remember not to get discouraged if you feel that your recovery
is taking a long time. Try to get through one day at a time and to make
progress in your recovery each day. Rest assured, within a few weeks or
months you will be feeling "back to normal"—and even better than you
ever felt before. And, in several months to a year, you will be able to
resume all of the activities you took part in prior to your surgery.

It is a good idea to ask *your* doctor for a "back-to-activity" schedule.
Your doctor will be able to tell you roughly when you can resume exercising, driving, going to school, working, carrying heavy objects, and so
on. As a general rule, you can trust your feelings when it comes to
resuming activity post-operatively. If you feel comfortable doing something—if it does not cause you pain or discomfort—then you will probably be relatively safe doing it. Still, you should pay attention to what
your doctor says. Too many times people have strained themselves after
surgery and, in doing so, broken their rods or harmed their fusions. Do
not be one of these people. Try to be as mindful of your spine, which
will need about six months to an entire year to fully fuse, as you are of
your desire to return to "life as usual."

PHYSICAL ACTIVITY DURING THE POST-OPERATIVE PERIOD

Physical activity is limited to walking for the first two to four weeks,
depending on levels fused, instrumentation, and brace use and type.
Thereafter, activities should be limited to gentle bending and moderate
lifting of a few pounds. Physical exercises such as isometrics, strength-
ening, and aerobic conditioning can begin four weeks after surgery for
most patients. Activity can be increased to include moderate household
and outdoor activities within four to six months for most adolescents.
In all of these, twisting and repetitive bending at the waist comes with
a caution for patients who have had significant portions of their lumbar spine fused. Full activity usually can happen within one year for

adolescents. Some patients may be excluded from certain contact sports (football, wrestling, soccer) and gymnastics indefinitely, depending upon number of levels fused and remaining flexibility. Good body mechanics is to be practiced for the long term. For patients fused to the lower thoracic spine, no restriction will be needed for the rest of their lives. For those fused to the lowest lumbar spine, moderate physical activity would be wise to lessen the impact of stress on remaining unfused joints in order to delay the degenerative process of aging.

FREQUENTLY ASKED QUESTIONS ABOUT SURGERY

◆ Is a clean air room used as it is for total joint replacements?
Most hospitals and surgeons don't use this for spinal surgery, as it is not necessary. It is not the standard of care.

◆ Are prophylactic antibiotics needed for procedures such as teeth cleaning as it would be for total joint replacements? Why (yes or no)?
This varies from doctor to doctor and is recommended for dental surgery, not general cleaning.

◆ Titanium vs. steel: What are the pros and cons?
Refer back to "Titanium vs. Steel" in this chapter.

◆ Will the rods have to be removed afterwards?
No, generally not.

◆ What percentage of rods needs to be removed?
Very small, less than one to four percent. In general, adolescents rarely have to have rod removal.

◆ What usually necessitates the need for rod removal?
Pain from prominence of the hardware, infection that can best be treated only by removal of the implant, especially in the late stages, or, in a very young child who is still growing and does not need to have the hardware remain during the growth period.

◆ Where will the bone be taken from for the fusion?
The ribs or the iliac crest.

◆ What are the risks of infection from a bone bank graft—specifically HIV and hepatitis?
Very small, less than 1:800,000.

◆ What are the sterilization processes?
Autoclave machine; gas sterilization.

◆ Does bone from the bank have a higher rate of nonunion (nonfusion)?
Bank bone by itself does not have a high union rate and is best used with the local bone or bone from the iliac crest, or ribs. When used exclusively, it may result in nonunion, especially in the lumbar spine and in adult patients.

◆ What are the benefits of using the bone bank?
Quantity—there is more bone volume for fusion, especially at multiple levels, if the patient does not have enough bone from the iliac crest or the rib(s). Patients who have had previous fusions, and have had bone grafts removed, may not have any reserve for additional grafting.

◆ What can the patient do beforehand to help increase the surgical and recovery outcome?
Exercise, maintain a positive attitude, do not smoke, practice respiration exercises, eat a good, balanced diet.

◆ How much loss of mobility is to be expected?
The lower down the lumbar fusion, the less mobility remains—the goal is always to preserve motion segments as much as possible to maintain spine balance and flexibility.

◆ The primary doctor performs the critical parts of operation. Who assists the doctor?
Residents and fellows, or another orthopedic surgeon.

◆ What are the precautions and monitoring devices used to ensure safety to the spinal cord?
Electrophysiological monitoring (SSEP), which monitors motor-

evoked potentials for posterior sensory column, and the classic wake-up test done at the end of surgery when anesthetic agents are lessened so the patient can be aroused and asked to move toes and feet.

◆ What is the risk of paralysis, and can it be corrected should it occur?
Very low in most cases, less than 1:1,000, being reported as .07%. It can be corrected if it is identified immediately and the offending process can be reversed, such as removal of instrumentation implant that may be causing pressure on the spinal elements, or reversal of the correction.

◆ During the operation, is a neurosurgeon part of the operating team?
A neurosurgeon is not usually part of the operating team for spinal deformity, unless there is a problem or a procedure needed to be performed on the spinal nerve roots.

◆ How is pain managed immediately post-operatively, in the following days, and the following weeks?
Morphine or Demerol can be administered intravenously or intramuscularly. Then, as the patient improves, oral medications such as Percocet, Vicodan, Tylenol III, and Darvocet are generally used. Subsequently, a mild analgesic, such as Tylenol is used.

◆ What are some of the late complications on the spine following surgery in the years to follow, since there is going to be greater stress on the remaining nonfused vertebrae?
A late complication is basically a degenerative process that is age-related on the remaining unfused segments. The lower one is fused in the lumbar spine, the greater likelihood of degenerative changes occurring in the remaining motion segments.

◆ If the patient has already lost some pulmonary function (before surgery), should pulmonary function testing be done pre-operatively?
Yes—for a baseline.

◆ Can there be any surgical complications or post-op pulmonary problems that need to be addressed?
Yes, pneumothorax, pleural effusion, pneumonia. (See "Risks and Benefits of Surgery" in chapter 4.)

◆ Should a pulmonologist be consulted with now, and should one be present during surgery in case of any problems?
A pulmonologist is not needed in surgery.

◆ Which patients are at risk for the crankshaft phenomena?
Children under ten years of age with a large curve exceeding sixty degrees are at risk.

◆ Can the spine continue to bend over the top of the rods (where it is not fused) after surgery?
Yes, a functional deformity can occur if the fusion is short or if the bone above is weak.

◆ Why might a doctor use bone bank graft instead of autologous bone from the ribs or hip?
Because there is not enough bone to obtain from the patient.

◆ In addition to the normal scoliosis standing X rays, bending films will also be taken prior to the surgery. If these films show a marked improvement in the curvature, will less of a fusion be considered?
Not really. Maybe only one curve will have to be fused; i.e., selective thoracic fusion. The more flexible, the more correction.

◆ Will there be any numbness around the incision after the surgery, and will the numbness diminish over time?
Yes.

◆ Will the rods set off the alarms at an airport? Is it a good idea to carry a note from the doctor if it will set off alarms?
Rods do not usually set off the alarm at the airport. Five to ten percent may, however. Patients are informed of this possibility, and they need to carry a card indicating that they have had spine surgery with instrumentation.

◆ What are the exercises to be done post-operatively by the patient? Is it better to know what is involved before the surgery to be familiar with them?
Isometric, transfer techniques, and aerobic conditioning with time. It's important to be familiar with good body mechanics.

◆ Do the scoliosis surgery and rods influence or compromise future pregnancies and deliveries?
Not at all. But epidural injection may be difficult or impossible if fusion extends to the lower lumbar spine.

◆ Are compression fractures less likely to occur? More likely? No difference? (This has to do with how the instrumentation and fusion relates to later osteoporosis.)
More likely in osteoporotic elderly patients, not in adolescents.

◆ How long is a typical hospital stay?
Five to seven days for posterior spinal fusion or anterior spinal fusion. Ten days to two weeks for a 2-stage anterior spinal fusion and posterior spinal fusion.

◆ What is the easiest type of curve to correct?
Single curve flexible thoracic or lumbar.

One last thing for you to remember after having surgery is that you have a right to see your operative report. If for any reason—or even for no reason at all—you ever want to see your operative report, your doctor is obliged to give you a copy of it. Some doctors are hesitant to do this; if your doctor refuses to give you an operative report from your surgery, be persistent in demanding it. The report will tell you exactly what went on in the operating room during your surgery and will describe the specifics of your surgery should you need to know them at any time in the future.

An Intimate Look at Surgical Experiences

ERIKA

After six tumultuous years of dealing with scoliosis, back braces, pain, decisions, and physical deformity, it was time. Erika was well-overdue for surgery. When she was thirteen, her thoracic curve had measured fifty degrees and her lumbar curve sixty-five. Doctors had, at that point, told Erika and her mother Denise that surgery was imperative. Over the course of the next year, Denise did extensive research on spinal fusions. She, like many other parents, had sought to find the best doctor, the best hospital, the best instrumentation system, the best surgical approach, and the best time of year for her daughter's operation. While Denise's research was in her daughter's best interest, the time it took was not. At fourteen, Erika had a thoracic curve measuring sixty degrees and a lumbar curve measuring seventy-four degrees. In addition to this lateral curvature, the rotation of Erika's spine had become so severe that it had begun to compromise her breathing and physical comfort. Erika was short of breath much too often, and the contorted back muscles her scoliosis had occasioned caused her both physical pain and aesthetic angst.

At the end of a long year of research and contemplation, Denise decided that Erika needed to have surgery immediately. She and Erika had chosen a hospital, a doctor, an approach, and a time for the surgery; it was to be a posterior spinal fusion done in late July 1997. Not only had Denise and Erika planned for Erika's scoliosis surgery, but they had spent much time and energy mentally preparing for it, which is why the sudden cancellation of the surgery a week before its scheduled date was so deeply disappointing.

The discouraging news arrived when Denise brought Erika to the hospital to have her pre-operative X rays taken. Upon seeing these X rays, Erika's surgeon noted that her spine had rotated significantly in the short time that had passed since her last set of X rays. In fact, Erika's spine had rotated so much that it had gone beyond anything her doctor had seen in his previous surgical experience. Due to this unexpected increase in rotation, Erika's doctor decided that he was not aptly qualified to perform the surgery Erika now required. He referred her to a doctor in Maryland, whose experience was more appropriate for Erika's current surgical needs.

"After we had psyched ourselves up so much and gotten ourselves mentally prepared for the surgery, it was so hard to be let down," Denise remembers. Erika had been very apprehensive about her imminent surgery; it had taken her so long just to convince herself that she could go through with it. Now that she had been delayed, she would have to go through the difficult mental preparation process all over again.

In August 1997, Erika and Denise traveled from Connecticut to Maryland to consult with Erika's new doctor. After examining Erika, he explained that he would do a joint anterior/posterior approach to the surgery. In other words, the doctor felt that Erika's scoliosis was severe enough to warrant both an anterior release (reaching the spine by way of the abdomen) of the spine and a posterior fusion (reaching the spine by way of the back) of the spine. Having explained this to Erika and Denise, the doctor in Maryland told them that he would be happy to do Erika's surgery; however, his first surgical opening was on September 23, three days before her fifteenth birthday. Potentially, there were many problems with this date: it would cause Erika to miss school that she had not planned to miss; it would put her in the hospital for her fifteenth birthday; and it would protract the emotionally draining, presurgical preparation.

"That's fine," Denise said, in response to the doctor's suggestion. "We'll do it then." Denise had originally planned for her daughter to have a simple, posterior spinal fusion in June 1997, at a hospital in Connecticut; now, Erika was to have a combined anterior/posterior spinal fusion on September 23, 1997, at a hospital in Maryland. The only reason why Denise ignored all of the downfalls that accompanied the new surgery plan was that she knew that Erika's need for surgery was becoming more urgent every day. Erika's scoliosis was progressing at such a rapid rate that she had to have the surgery as soon as possible; and, if an appointment in Maryland for September 23 was the best and quickest surgery option doctors could offer Erika and Denise, they would take it—regardless of any inconveniences or qualms they had with it.

The preparation for Erika's *real* surgery—the second one she and her mother had planned—began in early August. At this time, the hospital in Maryland suggested that Erika begin donating blood for the autologous blood transfusion she would need during surgery; the doctor and hospital staff estimated that Erika would need about six units of blood. Since Erika, who is anemic, preferred not to donate her own blood, she asked some close friends and family members with her same blood type to donate blood for her.

Having taken care of most of the presurgical preparations in Maryland, Denise and Erika returned home to Connecticut until September. They arrived back in Baltimore on a Sunday, two days before the day of surgery, and settled in at the local Ronald McDonald House, which welcomed families of patients at the nearby hospital. On Monday morning, Erika left the Ronald McDonald House and departed for the hospital, where she had her blood and vital signs tested and endured some presurgical neurological examinations.

In addition to performing these tests on Erika, the hospital personnel put her on oral antibiotics to ward off any remnants of a recent flu-like illness she was experiencing and concluded that it would be all right to proceed with Erika's plans to have surgery. That night, Erika's mother and grandmother took Erika out to the local Hard Rock Cafe for dinner as a special presurgery treat. After dinner, the three returned promptly to the Ronald McDonald House so that Erika could get a good night's sleep before her surgery.

Soon, Tuesday morning dawned. Erika, her mother, and her grandmother rose early and made their way to the hospital by 6:30 A.M. To Denise's relief, Erika was completely rid of her fever that day and felt ready for her operation. Upon her arrival at the hospital, Erika was asked to change from her street clothes into a hospital gown. Once Erika had changed, a nurse gave her an injection of Valium to relax her. The nurse then asked Denise to braid Erika's long, dark hair so that it would be out of the surgeon's way during the operation. As Denise followed this order, the Valium slowly began to have an effect on Erika; by the time Denise had finished braiding Erika's hair, she saw that her daughter was "almost completely out of it." Soon afterwards, nurses wheeled Erika's bed into the operating room.

As Erika's bed drew closer to the operating room, the hospital staff quickly handed Denise some scrubs to wear so that she would be allowed to walk into the holding area—the area right outside the operating room—and to say goodbye to her daughter. Denise kissed Erika and wished her good luck, then watched as the hospital staff wheeled her into the operating room. Denise broke down and began to cry.

"I couldn't be strong anymore," she admits. The stress brought on by the prospect of surgery, the maternal concern felt when one's child is being wheeled into an operating room, the reality that the time for surgery had actually arrived, and the apprehension about what would happen in that operating room finally crumbled her emotional stronghold. After years of discussion and lamentation about this scoliosis, the time for surgery had finally come.

Denise hails the hospital staff as being very informative throughout the surgery. The doctor performing Erika's surgery periodically sent envoys to the waiting room to keep Denise informed. Denise received notice when the doctor had made the anterior incision and had reached Erika's spine; when the doctor was halfway through with the anterior section; when he was closing the anterior incision; when the surgical team was turning Erika's body over to prepare for the posterior section; and so on. Throughout Erika's surgery, the hospital staff and the information they imparted was "very comforting" to Erika's family.

Just six and a half hours after Denise had seen her daughter wheeled into the operating room, she received notice that the entire surgery—including both the anterior *and* posterior sections—had been completed successfully. From the operating room, Erika was transferred to PICU (the Pediatric Intensive Care Unit). Erika was watched closely and received excellent care for the next twenty-four hours. Then she was removed from intensive care.

From that point on, Erika, in addition to Denise, was vigilant when it came to her care. Erika was persistent in asking doctors and nurses exactly what medication they were giving her, in what amount, and in what intervals. Despite her weakness from the surgery, she was intensely determined to make sure that there were no mishaps in her care.

For the seven total days and nights that Erika was in the hospital, Denise did not sleep. Following her stay in PICU, Erika began to have trouble with her bowels. *(Note: This problem is common in patients whose surgeries require long periods of anesthesia.)* Since Erika's bowels had been inert for six and a half hours, they had difficulty moving again. This is mostly due to the effects of narcotics and inactivity. Erika was treated with laxatives throughout the week, and when her bowels finally began to move, her doctor deemed her ready for discharge from the hospital.

At her home in Connecticut, Erika's family had created a makeshift bedroom for her on the first floor. For the first month of her recovery, though, Erika never used that room, because she could not lay flat. Instead, she slept in a large, reclining chair. After the first month, Erika began to sleep in the first-floor bedroom her family had made for her. And two months after her surgery, she was able to return upstairs to her own bedroom.

In November, Erika started a homebound tutoring program her school had arranged for her (all public schools are obliged to do this if their students need it). Homebound tutoring was the perfect solution to all of her postsurgery schooling needs. For the first month of this tutoring program, Erika found reading and working to be difficult due to the discomfort she was experiencing. When she started to feel better, though, Erika did very well with her studies.

The remainder of Erika's recuperative period was, according to Denise, "very eventful," but she weathered any difficulties she had quite well. Erika's and Denise's only complaint to date is that there is a slight protrusion of the surgical instrumentation in the lumbar-sacral area of Erika's spine. Though it does not cause Erika any pain, the protrusion is visible and, therefore, a point of concern from a cosmetic point of view.

Today, although Erika's spine is fused anteriorly from the T10 vertebra to the L4 vertabra and posteriorly from the T4 vertebra to the L4 vertebra (almost her entire spine), she is able to bend down and touch her toes. She returned to school long ago and has since been busy with friends, theater, and bike riding. Erika has not returned to playing any contact sports yet, although she would like to play softball.

In retrospect, Erika says that she would "do it [the surgery] over again" if she had to. Despite the many doubtful times, painful moments, and other difficulties that arose during and after her surgery, Erika is glad to have gone through with it. At fifteen years of age, she no longer has to worry about her scoliosis; she can, instead, revel in the fact that her spine is essentially straight and enjoy a life free from pain, deformity, and pulmonary problems.

"Before her surgery," Denise recalls, "Erika did not want to know much of anything about scoliosis or the surgical methods used to treat it. She was frightened by what was going to happen to her in the operating room and thought it would be better not to know about it."

Now, Erika attends meetings of a local scoliosis support group every month. Her curiosity about her condition has blossomed, and she is no longer afraid to learn about the disorder or its complications. She is proud to have gotten through surgery herself, and is always eager and willing to counsel others about scoliosis, to share her own experience, and to show her "battle scars." In addition to her postsurgical interest in scoliosis is Erika's new appearance. After her surgery, Erika decided, on her own, to cut her hair and lighten it to its natural shade of brown. Her new hairstyle accompanies a much more outgoing personality, which emanates from her smiling, easily visible face and her sparkling brown eyes. After years of battling scoliosis, fifteen-year-old Erika emerged a happy, healthy teenager—and the victor of the fight.

Denise's Recommendations for Parents of Children Having Surgery

- *Stay with the patient in the hospital at all times. (This varies from hospital to hospital. Be around, but not too vigilant.)*
- *Ask questions; make sure everything is taken care of.*
- *Make sure the hospital staff knows that a transfer has taken place (if your son or daughter has been transferred).*

- *Make sure the hospital staff has made the patient comfortable and has correctly connected all of the necessary tubes and intravenous fluids.*
- *Drinking (or otherwise receiving) fluids is important in helping the patient's bowels "wake up" and begin moving after the surgery—otherwise, the patient will have much discomfort. (Physical movement and reducing narcotics also helps.)*

JENNIFER

Four days after her surgery, fourteen-year-old Jen sat in the hospital cafeteria enjoying a Reese's peanut butter cup sundae. The hospital staff had wanted her to stay on a bland diet because she had been vomiting a lot from all the medicine she had been taking, but when her appetite returned, all Jen craved was an ice cream sundae. Her parents, who had taken her to the cafeteria, were so happy that Jen was in the mood to eat that they overlooked the hospital staff's advice and gave in to Jen's wishes. Contrary to what the hospital staff would have predicted, that Reese's peanut butter cup sundae ended up being the first food Jen was able to "keep down" after her surgery. Eating the forbidden but delicious sundae was a turning point for Jen; after she had devoured it, she felt considerably better than she had in previous days and felt as though she was on the road to recovery.

A few weeks prior to her eating the sundae, Jen had arrived at the hospital for the first time. That day, Jen began donating her blood so that the hospital would be able to give her autologous blood transfusions during her surgery.

"I was knocked out for the whole day," Jen remembers. "Giving blood was one of the worst parts of the whole surgery for me because I don't like needles."

Though having Jen give her own blood was optional and not required, Jen's mother, Jane, felt that "just to be on the safe side" Jen, herself, should donate the blood that would be used during her surgery. But after Jen had donated her first unit of blood, the hospital staff had told her she was anemic. This news did not come as a surprise to Jen or her mother; Jen had always been anemic. The single unit of blood she had already donated was all right to use, the hospital staff said, but Jen would definitely have to start taking iron pills before giving her next donation.

"The iron pills didn't agree with Jen," Jane says, "but she took them faithfully." One week after her first donation, Jen returned to the hos-

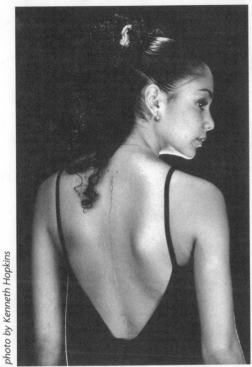

photo by Kenneth Hopkins

Jennifer three weeks after her surgery

pital to donate her second unit of blood.

As it turned out, Jen was never even able to donate her second unit of blood. When she returned to the hospital a week after her first donation—a week before the surgery—to give her second unit, the hospital staff found that her blood count was dangerously low, despite her having taken the iron pills. In fact, the hospital personnel informed Jen and her mother that, for a lack of blood to transfuse into Jen, and for Jen's fragile, anemic state, they might have had to postpone her surgery. This news jolted both Jen and Jane; they did not, under any circumstance, want to postpone Jen's surgery.

"When you're pumped up and ready to go through this [the surgery], you don't want it to be postponed for any reason," Jane explained.

Jen had never been worried about having surgery. She is not the type of person who had to calm her nerves or to mentally prepare herself for the surgery before having it. In fact, Jen *wanted* to have the surgery. After two years of brace wear, at the age of twelve, Jen had become fed up with her back brace. Therefore, at the age of twelve, Jen had decided to let her scoliosis go; she would allow it to progress until it required surgery. Then she would have the surgery, and be done with her scoliosis. Unlike many girls her age who are squeamish about surgery, Jen approached it with an air of fearless acceptance. She was the one who had chosen to have surgery; surgery was not the one who had chosen her. And now, at the age of fourteen, she was ready to come to terms with the choice she had made just two years ago.

Despite her not being tense about the surgery, Jen did not want to

postpone it. She wanted neither to unnecessarily drag out the preparation process she had been enduring for the past couple of weeks, nor
to put her family through the emotional agony of having to wait any
longer for this surgery to take place. Jen and her family would do anything they could to ensure that her surgery would occur on the scheduled surgery date.

When the news that Jen's anemia made her unable to donate any
more of her own blood arrived, the immediate reaction of Jen's mother and father was to donate their blood. But when Jen's parents proposed using their own blood for Jen's surgery, the hospital staff told
them that it was too late. The surgery date was too near at hand, and
Jen's parents' blood would not be returned to the hospital from the
screening and cleansing center in time for the surgery.

Now there were only a few days remaining before the surgical date. Jen
and Jane had to make a decision as to whether or not Jen was going to
have the surgery then. Jen would only be able to have the surgery under
two conditions: one, there would have to be at least two (preferably
more) units of blood ready to transfuse into Jen if she needed it during the
surgery; and two, Jen would have to take enough iron pills to get her blood
count up to a level at which it would be safe for her to undergo surgery.

Jen's family overcame the first obstacle by consenting to have Jen
transfused with the hospital's supply of blood—from anonymous
donors—if she needed extra blood during the surgery.

"We researched it and found out that the blood banks are pretty
safe now," Jane says. "They screen the blood very well." Once they had
allayed their fears regarding the blood donation supply, they moved on
to conquer the next obstacle: Jen's blood count.

"We got her all set with iron and gave her stuff to take that really got
her blood count up," says Jane. By the time the day for surgery had
arrived, Jen had a much higher blood count. The hospital deemed her
ready to have the surgery.

Day One (at the hospital): Jen arrived at the hospital at seven in the
morning—an hour before her scheduled surgery. After she had changed
into a hospital gown, she was situated on a moveable hospital bed and
prepared to go into the operating room. Jen remembers that a nurse
asked her whether she wanted to have her anesthesia via a mask or an IV.

"I chose the IV but they ended up giving me the mask, anyway," Jen
says, looking confused.

"Jen doesn't really remember this part," Jane explains. "They got her started with the IV to ease her into falling asleep. At the very end, she was still kind of awake in the operating room, so they decided to give her the gas, too."

Because the anesthesia that had been administered to her had already clouded her consciousness by the time her hospital bed was wheeled into the operating room, Jen has no memory of what went on from the time she bid her mother goodbye to the time when her surgery was complete.

For the next several hours Jane sat patiently in the hospital waiting room, waiting to hear news of progress in Jen's surgery. The doctor performing Jen's surgery sent someone out into the waiting room every half hour throughout the surgery to keep Jane abreast of what was happening in the operating room.

"Initially, they had told me that the surgery would only take four to six hours," says Jane. "They told us when they were putting the hooks in; they said they were putting the rods in after about seven hours; and after about eight hours, they told us that they were starting to put the bone graft on Jen's spine. After nine hours, they were finally finished."

When, during the surgery, Jane asked a nurse why it was taking so long, she received no answer. Even later, when she and Jen inquired about the length of time the surgery had taken, their doctor did not give them a direct answer. Disregarding the length of time it took, though, Jen's surgery was very successful. After the whole ordeal Jen and her family had gone through to arrange a blood supply for the surgery, Jen's doctor ended up transfusing her with the single unit of blood that she, herself, had donated. It turned out that Jen bled very little during the surgery and that the cell saver—a machine that automatically extracts lost blood, processes it, and recycles it as new, transfusable blood—provided Jen with all of the extra blood she needed in addition to the single unit.

At 5:00 P.M. on the day of her surgery, Jen was wheeled into the Pediatric Intensive Care Unit with a straight spine and almost no recollection of anything that had happened that day. Her breathing tube was still in place at that point, and her doctor had to perform the standard "wake-up test" on Jen before removing it. Drawing Jen just barely out of her anesthetic slumber, the doctor asked her to wiggle her hands and her toes. When she accomplished these minor feats, the doctor knew that she was conscious and that it would be all right to remove the breathing tube and to let Jen breathe on her own. The insertion and removal of the breathing tube down her throat had been Jen's biggest pre-surgical fears; luckily, she remembered neither episode once she was fully conscious. The only reminder Jen had of the removal of her breathing tube was the resulting incredibly sore throat. When she complained of having a sore throat, her doctor told her that it was nothing to worry about and that it was a very common aftereffect of having had a breathing tube.

After having removed Jen's breathing tube, her doctor placed an oxygen mask on her and situated her in her bed in the Intensive Care Unit. Shortly after Jen had been settled, her family was allowed to visit her.

"When we came to see her [Jen] right after the surgery," Jane says, "the scariest thing was that she was very swollen because she had been on her stomach for nine hours during the surgery. Her face was swollen—her eyes and lips—everything. And her hands and feet were huge and hard."

"I remember looking at my feet and saying, 'Oh my God!'" says Jen. "I didn't realize that my face was swollen also."

Concerned as to why her daughter appeared to be so distended, Jane asked a nurse in ICU why Jen had become so swollen. The nurse answered that most of Jen's swelling was a result of her blood having rushed to her face while she was on her stomach during surgery; she assured Jane that, with the help of Velcro wraps around Jen's body, the swelling would go down in the next few days. The Velcro wraps the nurse was referring to resembles the cuff wrapped around your arm when a doctor takes your blood pressure. They were wrapped around Jen's bloated legs for about four days, alternately tightening and loosening every few minutes to keep the blood actively flowing through all parts of her body.

"They were so annoying," Jen says of the wraps around her legs. "They kept me up during the night." Despite their being annoying, the Velcro wraps kept Jen's blood flowing and ultimately decreased the swelling of her body, so she was grateful for them.

Day Two: Jen had slept well during her first night in the hospital. The hospital staff had increased the amount of morphine administered overnight because they knew that they would be transporting her out of ICU the next day. The transport out of ICU would probably cause Jen more pain than had been experienced thus far, because she had not really moved since she had settled into ICU.

The morning after her surgery, Jen awoke with several IVs still attached to her body. Most of the IVs provided her with antibiotics; one gave her nutrient fluids to take the place of food, because she was not yet eating, and one supplied the morphine for her pain. Her supply of available, self-administered morphine was calibrated so Jen could push the button and give herself a dosage as often as every six minutes.

That morning, Jen was supposed to be transported from ICU, downstairs to the X-ray room, and then back upstairs to the adolescent unit of the hospital. Because of a miscommunication between hospital staff members, though, Jen was transported directly from the Intensive Care Unit to the adolescent unit on the same floor. Upon discovering that Jen had not had her post-operative X rays taken yet, the apologetic staff removed Jen from her bed in the adolescent unit and transported her downstairs to the X-ray unit. All of this unnecessary moving caused Jen a lot of pain; the doctors and nurses treating her knew this and, accordingly, increased her morphine dosage even more.

"They upped the morphine, and Jen was completely out," Jane remembers. "I was glad at that point to see her out of it, because otherwise she would have been so uncomfortable lying on that X-ray table."

Shortly after Jen had returned from the X-ray room to her room in the adolescent unit, a representative from an orthotist's office came to visit her. This woman unexpectedly arrived in Jen's room and began to take her measurements. Jen's doctor had apparently ordered a post-surgical back brace for Jen to wear. When Jen, who had been under the impression that she was not going to have to wear a brace after surgery, asked her doctor about the matter, he said that he had *just* decided to put her into a brace. He hadn't thought that he would need to do so before the surgery, but afterward, he had concluded that it would be a good idea to put Jen into a brace to ensure her support and protection during the first few months that her spine was fusing.

Day Three: Jen remembers feeling about ninety percent better on her third day. Despite her feeling better, though, Jen found her third day to be her most challenging. She did not feel ready to work with the hospital's physical therapist.

"I knew I couldn't get up," Jen says. Because of her having been under anesthesia so long during the surgery, it had been especially difficult for Jen to start feeling clearheaded, awake, and "normal." She had been lying completely flat for two days; even the slightest movement of her hospital bed toward a sitting position made her dizzy. Nevertheless, Jen's doctor and nurses thought that it was time for Jen to start moving, so they called the physical therapist to her room.

The physical therapist entered Jen's room and just sat her up, thinking that helping Jen would be very easy. No one can blame the physical therapist for having assumed this; in most cases, post-operative spine fusion patients are very reluctant to start physical therapy, but once they begin, they feel energized and start to recover remarkably quickly. Unfortunately, this was not the case with Jen; her reluctance to sit up was genuine. When the physical therapist pushed her body into a sitting position, Jen started to hyperventilate.The physical therapist eased her back down into a supine position and agreed to "give her another day" before moving ahead with any more physical therapy. Jane remembers that the few minutes Jen spent with the physical therapist "knocked her out" for the remainder of that day. Jen still had not regained her appetite, and she had not eaten since before her surgery. She therefore had almost no energy, and small exertions like her brief encounter with the physical therapist could exhaust her for an entire day.

Also, on Jen's third day, her nurses took her off morphine, replacing it with a different pain-killing drug called Percocet. But because Jen had not eaten for so many days, she did not react well to the Percocet and became nauseous. She worried about vomiting. But she had no need to worry; the hooks and rods had been secured well amidst her vertabrae, and they stayed in place throughout her sickness and her recovery.

Day Four: Jen's fourth day at the hospital happened also to be the Fourth of July. By this time, Jen was feeling almost one hundred percent better. Her physical therapist had come into her room in the morning and had helped her to begin walking by herself, so that by the afternoon, Jen was eager to get up and walk around.

"I wanted to get up and go to the bathroom by myself," Jen remembers. "I couldn't stand using that bedpan anymore." Her parents asked her if she wanted them to wheel her to the cafeteria (she was not yet strong enough to walk all the way there) and, to their surprise, Jen agreed to go. It was at that point that she dismissed her nurses' sanctions and her own inhibitions and dared to eat a Reese's peanut butter cup sundae. And from that moment on, she was eating again and feeling ready to go home.

That night, Jen welcomed her friends who had come to the hospital to visit her. She felt "almost normal" again, and was happy to talk with her friends as she walked around the hospital's teen activity center with them. Though Jen did not go out to see any fireworks that Fourth of July, she was able to see the Fourth of July fireworks through her hospital window. She fell asleep watching the aerial bursts of red, white, and blue, knowing that she would soon be going home.

After her fifth day at the hospital, Jen returned home. Jen found that she was physically unable to take part in much activity during her first few days home; she suffered from lethargy and some pain, and she had not completely gained her appetite back. Moreover, Jen did not *want* to do much of anything. She did not feel like taking part in activities or going out with friends; all she wanted to do was to lie at home and relax.

"I didn't want to go out at all because I didn't want to wear the back brace," she says, candidly. Jen knew that if she stayed safely at home, she would have no need for the protection and support the brace provided; whereas if she went out, she would certainly need the support of the back brace. Since Jen was afraid to venture outside of her house *without* the brace on, yet she absolutely did not want to wear the brace, she simply did not go out.

"Jen needed to hear from the doctor that she wasn't going to ruin the surgery by not wearing the brace," Jane says. "When we saw the doctor after Jen's release from the hospital, he assured her that the brace was mainly for her protection and support. He said a lot of people feel more confident with it on, but that he understood it wasn't going to be easy for her to wear it."

Jen's doctor suggested that she wear the brace while in the car or if she was going to be somewhere where there was a crowd for the first couple of weeks following her surgery. He did not want to risk having Jen banged, jolted, or bumped into during the time that her spine was just beginning to fuse.

"Jen would wear the brace in the car," Jane says, "but she would take it off even before she got out of the car. I guess she figured that she had gone through all of that [the surgery] just so that she wouldn't have to wear a brace. So now, she kind of had a right not to wear one."

Although her own body and attitude—and not someone else's reservations—were mainly responsible for physically and socially inhibiting her post-operatively, Jen resented her situation at times. Being home all the time dragged her spirits down, and she expressed a lot of doubt about having gone through with the surgery. Day by day, though, as her body and spirit advanced in the healing process, Jen became happier with her decision to have had the surgery. As she gathered strength and began to feel like herself again, Jen became proud of what she had accomplished, and any traces of regret vanished.

The turning point in Jen's recovery was the day she ventured outside to watch her softball team's last game of the season; it was the only game Jen had missed, and she had to miss it because of her surgery.

"I had my last softball game, and I couldn't play in it," she says. "That's when I went out, when I went to go watch my softball game. We went to my friend's house and had a cookout afterwards. And after that day, I was pretty much going out."

Today, Jen's life resembles her life prior to surgery. Instead of worrying about her scoliosis, she is thinking about starting high school in the fall; instead of being depressed about surgery-related pain and fatigue, she is excited about the fact that her spine will have fused completely by the time the next softball season rolls around.

There *are* a few differences in Jen's life now, and most apply to her appearance. In addition to having gained the thin scar that runs over a foot in length down her back, Jen has gained a lot of physical symmetry as a result of her surgery. Jane has noticed that, whereas one of Jen's "chicken bones" shoulder blades [scapulas] protruded more than the other before, they are now even. And the one shoulder that was always a little bit higher than the other now appears to be balanced with the other.

Three weeks after her surgery, there are still some areas of Jen's back that are numb; this is a result of some nerves having been cut during the surgery. But the nerves will grow back, and for the time being, Jen does not miss them. All she cares about is the fact that her spine, once curved forty-eight degrees, is now curved only nineteen degrees. When Jen and Jane saw the X rays of Jen's straightened spine, they marveled at them.

"I didn't expect it [the spine] to look like that," Jen says. After having looked at X rays of a crooked spine for so many years, one can imagine how unbelievable it is to see an X ray of the same spine after it has been straightened. The X ray is proof to both Jen and Jane that their physical and emotional stress during and after the surgery was worth their while. Both mother and daughter can rest assured that Jen's struggle with scoliosis is finally over.

Jennifer's and Jane's Recommendations for People Having Surgery
- *Plan the blood donations ahead of time. If the patient cannot give his or her own blood, have his or her parents' blood checked and donated several weeks in advance.*
- *You lose a lot of weight during and after the surgery due to loss of appetite, so don't be afraid to gain five to ten pounds in the weeks or months leading up to the surgery; you'll benefit yourself by gaining some weight beforehand. (Be sure to consult with your doctor and nutritionist.)*
- *The patient's face and body may be very swollen after surgery—especially if the surgery takes several hours; don't worry, the swelling will soon go down.*
- *If you are a parent, stay with your child throughout his or her recovery. Don't nag or ask your child too many questions, but make sure that everything is being done to make him or her comfortable and to expedite the recovery process. (Communicate with your doctor about your child's recovery process.)*

ANTHONY

When Anthony's orthopedic doctor moved from Connecticut to North Carolina, Anthony was automatically paired with the new doctor who had taken his previous doctor's position at the hospital. The new doctor had never met Anthony, yet upon examining him for the first time, he felt that he knew enough about Anthony's case to draw an immediate conclusion.

"You need surgery," the doctor said to Anthony, a seventeen-year-old high school senior with a fifty-one-degree thoracic curve. "You need to have it right away, even before this school year is over, and you probably won't be able to graduate with your class." Anthony knew from that moment that he did not like this new doctor.

"He was devastated," Anthony's mother, Pat, remembers. "He forgot about the brace he had been wearing and refused to address the issue of his scoliosis."

Anthony was very unhappy with and unresponsive to the new doctor at the hospital. He felt that the doctor had an unnecessarily blunt approach and a poor bedside manner. Knowing that they could not just dismiss what this doctor had said, Anthony's parents contacted his pediatrician, who referred them to another scoliosis specialist.

This new doctor had a much gentler demeanor. He was professional, honest, and straightforward; yet he managed to integrate genuine feeling and a real concern for Anthony's well-being and lifestyle into his diagnosis. To Anthony's dismay, this doctor also recommended that he have surgery. When the previous doctor had spouted this diagnosis, Anthony had been skeptical about it; now, though, Anthony knew that surgery was a reality that he would have to face.

His new doctor respected the fact that Anthony wanted to complete his senior year before having surgery, but warned Anthony and his parents that if they waited too long, the scoliosis would begin to adversely affect his heart and lungs. Though Anthony's lateral curvature was only fifty-one degrees—making him an apt but not an urgent surgical candidate—the rotation of his spine was substantial and would, in the future, compromise Anthony's heart function and lung capacity.

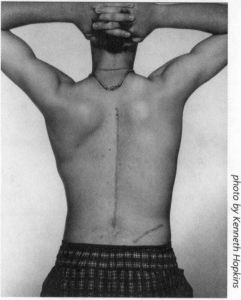

photo by Kenneth Hopkins

Anthony four months after surgery exhibiting scars on his back and on his hip, the site of bone graft removal.

Having accepted that Anthony would have to have surgery for his scoliosis, Anthony's family took time to digest the news. For two months, they talked to friends, other family members, and people on the Internet about Anthony's situation. Once the holiday season had passed and Anthony had turned eighteen, his parents knew that it was time to make a decision. Until this day, Anthony's parents maintain that the decision to let Anthony have this elective surgery was one of the most difficult decisions they have ever had to make. Despite their difficulty making the decision, Anthony and his parents reluctantly scheduled surgery for April—just two months before Anthony was to graduate from high school.

In February, Anthony began to take iron pills to make sure that he had a high blood count before he gave his pre-surgery autologous blood donations. He donated two units of blood on March 8, and two units on March 22. The week before his surgery, Anthony visited the hospital to register, fill out paper work, and get his blood work done. At that point he was asked to choose whether he wanted to register as an adult patient or as a child; Anthony registered as an adult, assuming that he would have an altogether quieter surgical experience if he was in the adult—as opposed to the pediatric—unit of the hospital.

Anthony was admitted into the hospital at 6:30 A.M. on the morning of his surgery. Amazingly, that morning, and throughout his entire surgical process, Anthony felt neither nervous nor scared. He had never been deterred or upset by the fact that he had to have surgery; what bothered him was the fact that having the surgery would keep him out of sports for a full year. Therefore, while most people are filled with anxiety on the morning of surgery, Anthony was relatively indifferent.

"It's just life," he said. "Why be nervous?" As he was wheeled into the operating room, his prevailing thought was, "whatever happens, happens." His parents—who were a lot more nervous than Anthony was— went to the waiting room at that point and began several hours of waiting. Throughout the surgery, nurses came out to the waiting room to keep Anthony's parents updated on what was happening in the operating room. And the entire time the surgery was taking place, Anthony's best friend, Michael, was at school watching the clock. With every minute that passed, Michael wondered how Anthony was doing and narrated to the other kids at school what was *probably* happening in the operating room at any given point.

In just a few hours, Anthony's spine had been straightened with titanium rods, which had just come on the market a month before. He had been transfused with two units of blood during the surgery, and everything had gone very well. The surgery had been successful, Anthony's spine was now straight, and Anthony and his parents were eager for Anthony to start his recovery soon.

Anthony knew that, after his surgery, his face would be swollen from all the anesthesia and from lying prone for so long. In the first days of his recuperation, therefore, he didn't mind his swollen appearance, though it bothered his family. To see Anthony lying there, completely swollen, with numerous IVs attached to him, was a sight difficult for Anthony's parents and siblings to see. Yet they knew that they had to be emotionally strong for Anthony during this recovery, so they tried not to let their own feelings of anxiety become apparent. They made plans to stay with Anthony around the clock. Never was there a moment during which Anthony was by himself. His family's devotion to helping him and their presence throughout his recovery helped Anthony regain his strength, get on his feet again, and leave the hospital in just four days.

Day One: After his surgery, Anthony was asked to rate his level of pain on a scale of one to ten. When he estimated that his pain was about a seven or an eight, nurses increased the amount of morphine that Anthony could administer to himself via a button at his bedside. Anthony pushed the morphine button so that he would feel less pain, and drifted off into a day-long slumber. Both the nurses tending to Anthony and Anthony's parents thought it was normal for Anthony to be sleeping this much after he had just had surgery. No one suspected that anything was wrong with Anthony until, suddenly, his eyes opened—as if he were waking up—and rolled back. Anthony's parents, who were sitting at his bedside, knew that this was not normal; when asked to wiggle his fingers as a sign that he was all right, Anthony could not lift his finger.

"He looked like he had awakened from a bad dream," his parents remember. Then, Anthony turned to his parents, looked at them, and managed to say, "I need help." Upon hearing this, Anthony's parents alerted nearby nurses. The nurses contacted the pain management team, who administered an antidote to counteract the morphine he had been taking. Anthony's reaction had been the result of a mild morphine overdose, but in a matter of minutes he was feeling better. *(Note: There should be a pulse oxymeter alarm to alert staff of such events. This is the normal procedure in recovery rooms.)*

Day Two: On the second day of his hospital stay, Anthony was feeling considerably better than he had felt immediately after the surgery. A physical therapist came to his room and was able to help Anthony to sit up, and then to get up, to walk to a chair, to sit in the chair, and to walk back to his hospital bed. Amazingly, Anthony was able to do all of this just a day after he had surgery! Later that day, he was ready for visitors.

At around noon, Anthony was in a full sitting position in his bed when his friends visited. Anthony felt "back to normal" after visiting with his friends. Luckily, his intrinsic determination and thirst for action and adventure would not permit him to remain in a hospital bed for very long.

Day Three: On his third day at the hospital, Anthony made even more progress with his physical therapist. With some help, he managed to walk down the hospital hallway and even to walk up and down some stairs. While Anthony's physical therapist was very impressed with the progress he was making, Anthony was never surprised by the sheer rapidity of his post-operative physical progress; he had known all along that his recovery would be a fast one and that he would be back to school, friends, and sports in as little time as possible. It was obvious to everyone at the hospital that Anthony's intensely determined attitude was responsible for his speedy recovery and prompt return to real life.

Day Four: Anthony was discharged from the hospital on the fourth day following his surgery. He took Extra Strength Tylenol (he found that this was the best at-home agent to control his post-operative pain) for the first ten days he was home; after that, any pain he felt was minimal. For six weeks, Anthony was homebound. In order to keep up with the rest of his class, though, Anthony had a homebound tutor. When he returned to school in late May, he was as prepared to finish high school as any of his classmates were. Luckily, the dreadful prophesy of Anthony's old doctor had been a fallacy; despite the fact that Anthony had undergone surgery, he *would* be able to graduate with his class.

Anthony did emerge from his home a few times during his recovery. Just two and a half weeks after he had surgery, he ventured to a local meeting of a scoliosis support group. Anthony was one of three speakers to talk about personal experiences with surgery that night. Through his detailed account of his hospital experience, he was able to shed light on surgery for those who were contemplating it. And just by virtue of being at the meeting two and a half weeks post-operatively, Anthony inspired everyone there by presenting the fact that it was entirely possible to bounce right back to real life after having a spinal fusion.

Three and a half weeks after his surgery, Anthony attended his senior prom. Though it would still be two and a half weeks before Anthony returned to classes, he felt that his senior prom was something that he just could not miss. He wore a tuxedo, danced until dawn, and had a great time with his friends—not once worrying about or being hindered by his spine.

In June, about two months after Anthony had been discharged from the hospital, he graduated with the Class of 1997. The Anthony who graduated was, in many ways, unlike the Anthony whom the high school had known for so many years. The new Anthony had a straight spine and was one and a half inches taller as a result of his surgery. He emanated a mature sense of self-esteem and had a new air of accomplishment.

In retrospect, Anthony says that the worst part of his hospital experience was "the tape they used to secure the IV's." To him, the feeling of tape being put on and taken off his body was more painful than his spine ever was. Anthony maintains that the worst part of his recovery was "not being able to play sports for one year after the surgery." Being detained from sports and other activities that he enjoys so passionately was torture for Anthony. As soon as one year had passed post-surgery, he went back to playing his favorite sports, diving off cliffs, and bungee jumping. Though Anthony's doctor (and I would imagine *anybody's* doctor) encouraged him *not* to play contact sports or to try any dangerous stunts, even after his post-surgical year without activity, Anthony could not listen. While he is mindful of his spine, he feels that he must also be mindful of his spirit, which irrevocably impels him to play soccer, hockey, and lacrosse, and to attempt all of the things that he loves to do.

ZOE

Zoe's surgery was scheduled to take place in August, and titanium implants had just been approved for the market in March. Having done extensive research on scoliosis, doctors, hospitals, instrumentation systems, and surgical methods, Zoe'e mother had made the decision to request traditional, stainless steel rods for Zoe. She had no particular misgivings about titanium rods; she merely felt that stainless steel rods had been in circulation for a much longer period of time and that they had a good, solid history of being successful in spine fusions.

When Zoe's mother asked her doctor if he would use stainless steel implants for her surgery, he gladly agreed, saying that the request was "no problem at all." And, although Zoe's parents never signed a contract saying that her surgery would be done with stainless steel rods, they assumed that their request would be respected.

One week before the day of Zoe's scheduled surgery, she was at the hospital having her pre-operative blood work done. It was a surprise to Zoe, her mother, and the nurse taking her blood sample to find that the level of iron in Zoe's blood was quite low. The nurse warned Zoe and her mother that if she did not have her iron level up by the time she was admitted for surgery, her doctor would not be able to perform the surgery.

Frantic that she only had a week to get her daughter's iron level up, her mother began thinking of ways in which she could infuse Zoe with iron. Every morning for the next week, Zoe ate liver for breakfast. One can imagine that liver would not be the breakfast choice of a thirteen-year-old, and Zoe was no exception to this rule. By the time Zoe's surgical date

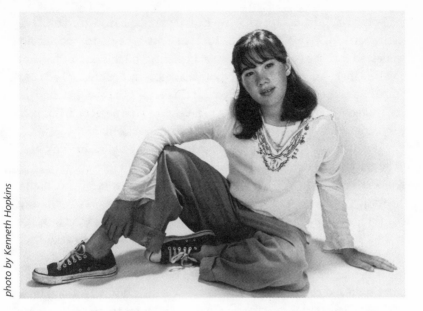

photo by Kenneth Hopkins

had arrived, her iron level had risen considerably, and she was in perfect condition to have the surgery. Both Zoe and her parents, while nervous about the surgery, were relieved that it did not have to be postponed.

Right before the surgery, Zoe's surgeon and his assisting surgeon spoke to Zoe's parents and told them that the entire operation—a basic posterior spinal fusion from the T4 vertebra to the L4 vertebra— would only take about four and a half hours to complete. Her parents were astonished when they heard this; they had expected to hear the doctors say that the surgery would take about eight hours. Nevertheless, they ventured into the hospital waiting room to begin their long period of waiting and parental anxiety.

When the periodic updates of Zoe's progress in surgery began coming, they were able to surmise that a mere four and a half hours would not suffice. Zoe's surgery would take more than eight hours, just as her parents had expected. Although her parents were updated as to what was going on in the operating room, they were never told why their daughter's surgery had taken so much longer than expected. At the end of eight hours, Zoe's surgeon came into the waiting room to report.

"He gave us a glowing report of the surgery and told us how successful the whole thing had been," her mother remembers. And after the doctor had assured Zoe's parents that everything had gone well and that Zoe was "great," he mentioned one detail about the surgery.

"By the way," the doctor said, "we had to use titanium instead of stainless steel rods." This infuriated Zoe's parents. They had specifically requested that she have stainless steel implants, and this doctor had not honored their request. When her mother asked why the doctor had used titanium against her wishes, the doctor told her that the rods planned for Zoe's surgery had been used during the night for an emergency. This provoked innumerable questions in the minds of Zoe's parents.

If the stainless steel rods had been used during the night, why hadn't the doctor obtained more stainless steel rods before starting Zoe's surgery? Why hadn't he informed Zoe and her parents of the instrumentation situation and allowed *them* to decide what they wanted to do? Had there only been one set of stainless steel rods in the hospital at the time of the so-called emergency? Was it necessary to take *Zoe's* rods? And why had the doctor waited so long to tell her parents about the fact that he was using titanium for Zoe? Rather than pursuing the point then and there, her parents expressed their discontent and let it go. They knew that they had to help their daughter through her recovery before confronting the doctor who had disregarded their wishes.

Zoe's only post-surgical problem was getting her bowels to move. After the entire body has been asleep for eight hours, it is often difficult to wake everything back up again. After her surgery, Zoe's bowel-related stomach pain caused her much more discomfort than her spine-related back pain ever did. Forcing all kinds of fluids and foods to rouse her digestive system received little response. But the doctors discharged Zoe five days after her surgery without her having had a bowel movement. Doctors do not normally discharge patients from the hospital until they have had post-surgical bowel movement, especially if the patient is having abdominal discomfort. But in Zoe's case, the hospital personnel came to the conclusion that Zoe's body would begin to function normally once she returned home, and they were correct. Upon Zoe's arrival at home, she was eating and drinking more, and she felt more relaxed and comfortable than she had in the hospital. She eventually had a bowel movement, and from that point on, she was on her way to feeling "normal" again.

A few weeks after she had undergone surgery, Zoe began the eighth grade. Over the summer, her spine had shifted from having a forty-one-degree thoracic curve and a fifty-one-degree lumbar curve to having a sixteen-degree thoracic curve and a twenty-two-degree lumbar curve; also, she had become one and a half inches taller. Though Zoe was excited to be starting school, she and her parents were concerned that the advent of the school year would bring rowdy kids and rough-housing in the hallways. This was a foreboding prospect to Zoe, who still felt fragile and as though she did not want her back to be touched. Zoe had not been braced after her surgery simply because post-surgical bracing was not recommended. Therefore, she felt especially vulnerable toward being hit or bumped into by accident when she was around people. To her relief, when Zoe returned to school, her peers were very gentle. They were very mindful not to push or bump into her, and their concern was much appreciated.

The only other school-related concern that Zoe and her parents had was "the book issue." She would be unable to carry a book bag for several months. Their solution was to get two sets of books for the year: one to keep at school, and one to keep at home. This way, Zoe had her books at her fingertips wherever she was, and she never had to carry a backpack or risk hurting her spine.

Though Zoe is fully recovered, active, and well, her parents remain focused on the fact that titanium is in her back.

Zoe's and Her Mother's Advice for People Having Surgery

- Make sure you know exactly what is going on in the operating room, and make sure the doctor listens to and acts on your suggestions and requests. *Any changes should be discussed.*
- Don't make any assumptions that what you want to happen will happen. If you want a particular instrumentation system to be used during surgery, your request and the doctor's promise to respect that request must be in writing.
- Two to three weeks post-operatively, begin putting vitamin E on your scar every night; the less vitamin E you apply, the more visible your scar will be.
- If you are a child or teenager who plans on returning to school shortly after your surgery, *do not* carry a book bag; keep one set of books at school, and obtain another set of books to keep at home.

The Annoyances that Accompany Surgery

- Having to give blood in intervals during the weeks leading up to the surgery.

- You have to refrain from participating in contact sports and performing demanding physical activity for one year after the surgery.
- Having to miss school or work while you recover.
- The fear of needles bothers many people more than the idea of the actual surgery.
- The sore throat resulting from the breathing tube used during surgery.
- Losing your appetite and losing weight for the first few days after surgery.
- Having to endure a brief X-ray session almost immediately following your surgery. *(Note: Most X rays are done while the patient is still asleep in the OR. Discharge X rays are done when the patient feels well standing.)*
- Being groggy from the pain medication you are given.
- Hospital food.
- Avoiding the sun after surgery—exposing your back to the sun will result in your scar permanently darkening.

THE BENEFITS OF HAVING SURGERY

- Most people "grow" an inch, or even a few inches, once their spines have been straightened; height gain varies from patient to patient.
- Knowing that, after much discussion, deliberation, and difficulty, your spine is finally straighter—the average correction is about sixty percent with current systems.
- Visits and assistance from friends and family.
- Your spine doesn't really even hurt afterwards (though the place where the doctor took the bone graft—either your rib or your hip—tends to hurt).
- Feeling victorious—as though you've conquered your scoliosis.
- Children and adolescents will no longer have to wear back braces.
- Getting rid of your cosmetic concerns—you may have a scar, but the rib hump is not prominent.
- You are in better health, and the risk of herniating a disc is reduced.
- Some kids are happy about missing school; those who are troubled by missing time at school can benefit from homebound tutoring.
- Although the actual surgery and recovery may prove to be a challenge, most people are ultimately "glad they did it."

THE RISKS OF HAVING SURGERY

◆ Pseudarthrosis, or nonunion, can occur for a number of reasons, including poor fusion technique, insufficient bone graft, decompensated lumbar curves and thoracolumbar curves in the adult, or infection. Long fusions to the sacrum treated posteriorly only and surgeries using non-segmental instrumentation can be more prone to this complication; chronic smoking can also exacerbate the risk. To reduce the risk of pseudoarthrosis, the doctor should do a thorough removal of all joints, using a large-enough bone graft or autogenous graft and segmental instrumentation. In the case of severe adult lumbar/lumbarsacral curve, you should consider anterior fusion, and of course, no matter what your surgical outlook, discontinue smoking.

◆ Neurologic paralysis or weakness can be caused by direct injury to neural structures or through excessive correction. Make sure the doctor plans a moderate, balanced correction based on flexibility.

◆ Infection due to wound contamination can be warded off by preoperative antibiotics; infection is more common in revision cases due to poor blood supply to tissue, so the doctor must use meticulous surgical technique to minimize the risk.

◆ Instrumentation failure can be caused by nonunion or inadequate fixation. Meticulous fusion-technique and segmental instrumentation can help ensure your instrumention works as it should.

◆ Decompensation can result from the failure to fuse a structural curve, the improper selection of fusion levels, or the addition on of a level after the initial fusion of a curve. Make sure your doctor fuses the structural major curve, fuses the entire curve, and selects fusion levels properly.

◆ Other complications and risks include pneumonia, blood clots, crankshaft effect (contour spine rotation after posterior fusion), and transufsion risks such as hepatitis. See the following chapter for more information on possible complications.

Chapter 6

Surgical Complications

Scoliosis surgery is like any other surgery in that you run the risk of experiencing certain complications. You can avoid some of these complications by listening to your doctor, knowing what you are allergic to, being careful not to strain yourself after surgery, practicing good eating and exercise habits before surgery, and being mindful of your spine and your general health. Still, there are some complications that you cannot avoid—some that you have absolutely no control over. The majority of scoliosis surgeries do not result in complications; those that *do* result in complications, though, cannot be denied.

If you run into a complication during or after your surgery, know that you are not alone and can recover from the complication. Many people have had complications in the past and, while these people remember the complications as having been physically and emotionally painful at the time, in retrospect most do not deem the complications to have been quite so difficult or important. Most of the time, complications are promptly corrected or treated. Some complications can leave a permanent deficit or disability, albeit rare.

ALLERGIC REACTION TO THE METAL IN YOUR IMPLANTS

Recently, many people have been found to be allergic to nickel, a metal component of the alloy known as stainless steel. Inserting stainless steel rods into the spines of people who are allergic to nickel can cause allergic reactions such as burning sensations, lesions, and rashes. Titanium (an alternative to stainless steel) implants are becoming more and more popular these days because titanium does not contain nickel and can, therefore, be used in the scoliosis surgeries of people who are allergic to nickel. If you are about to have surgery, find out whether you are allergic to nickel; know what your body is allergic to and what it is tolerant of before putting anything into it.

Unfortunately, some people, unaware of any sensitivity to nickel, have stainless steel instrumentation implanted into their spines. Allergic reactions begin to surface post-operatively. In such cases, the only thing to do is to have the rods removed. If the fusion has taken place, it is safe to simply have the rods removed and to leave the spine instrumentation-free. If the fusion has not taken place, doctors can replace the old instrumentation system with a new one (most likely titanium) to allow the spine to fuse in the *absence* of any bothersome allergic reactions.

SHERRY

Several months after her scoliosis surgery, Sherry began to see and feel changes in her back. She remembers having noticed "burning rashes like shingles" and "lesions the size of quarters." These lesions increased in size as Sherry's pain increased in intensity. Then, one day,

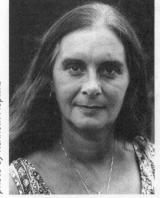

photo by Kenneth Hopkins

Sherry's daughter, Amanda, saw blood stains on her mother's clothing.

"Mommy, you're bleeding," said Amanda to Sherri. It was at this point that Sherry knew that something was definitely wrong with her back and that she needed to see a doctor. Sherry visited an immunologist allergist, who decided to test her for allergies. This specialist contacted the company that manufactured the rods used in Sherry's surgery and requested a test piece of the relevant stainless steel. Having obtained a sample of the stainless steel used in Sherry's rods, the specialist taped it to Sherry's back and asked her to keep it there for forty-eight hours. Forty-eight hours later, there was a quarter-sized, bleeding lesion on the skin beneath the sample of stainless steel. This test confirmed that Sherry was allergic to her implants—or, more accurately, to the nickel in her implants.

The only thing Sherry could do was to have her rods removed. The nickel in her body was causing her more pain than her scoliosis surgery had.

DECOMPENSATION

Decompensation is a deformity that is classified as progressive. This happens when the spine continues to curve above or below the fused levels, usually in the post-operative period of a primary surgery. This occurs "when the head (and/or trunk) doesn't line up over the center of the pelvis."[28] In younger people, this can best be treated by wearing a brace. In the adult, treatment means further surgery to extend the initial fusion.

FLATBACK

A flatback deformity is classified as an acquired deformity, or one that may occur after a surgical correction of a primary deformity. This refers to the loss of the natural curves in the back; namely, lumbar lordosis. This deformity has been known to be a common complication resulting

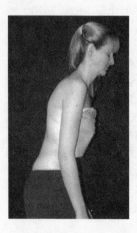 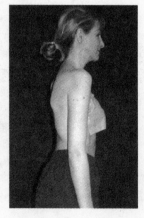

Left: Typical posture of a patient with postsurgical flatback deformity.

Right: Post-operative photo of the same patient. Note improvement in standing posture.

from the implantation of the Harrington Rod Distraction System, popular in the 1960s. It occurs because of the distraction of the system across the lumbar vertebrae. Gradually, the patient will present as "tilting forward." As degeneration progresses, muscles become weakened and patients become fatigued. "The classic presentation is an inability to stand erect with the knees straight."[29]

DRUG REACTIONS

Drug reactions and complications are common hazards of surgery. Take every precaution to review both the administration of any drugs and all the possible side effects. Be particularly sensitive to the possibility of morphine overdose after surgery. Make sure you're not allergic or overly sensitive to any of the pain killers before they are administered.

PSEUDARTHROSIS—FAILURE OF FUSION

Pseudoarthrosis means breakage of a fusion or failure of fusion to take place; this often happens when there are spinal implants. When there is a failure of fusion to take place, your spine is weaker and dependent on the implants. Additional surgery might be necessary.

PNEUMOTHORAX

Though pneumothorax sounds scary, it is easily treatable. It happens when air becomes trapped in the thoracic cavity. This can be an air leak from a punctured lung, or outside air trapped during open thoracotomy or thoracoplasty. This complication is rare and occurs most frequently during anterior surgery, rib resections with sharp rib edges, or violation of the pleura (a thin sheet of tissue covering the chest cavity) by a hook or part of a rod.

ROD BREAKAGE

A small percentage of people are afraid of rod breakage and have their rods taken out as soon as their spines are fused. This is unnecessary.

Rod breakage sometimes occurs while skiing, ice skating, falling, water skiing, or picking up something. Some people decide, through consultation with the doctor, to just live with the broken rod; others have the rod removed and hope that the fusion has taken place.

CRANKSHAFT EFFECT

This phenomenon can occur when a skeletally immature patient has a spinal fusion with metal rods. The surgery thwarts the growth of the fused backsides of the vertebrae while the front parts of the vertebrae continue to grow. The uneven growth pattern results in additional spinal deformation. A patient with a low Risser number combined with a large curve of over sixty degrees should consider this risk.

Some Complication Statistics

Pseudarthrosis—5 to 27 percent
Residual pain—5 to 15 percent
Pulmonary embolism (blockage of a blood vessel)—1 to 20 percent
Mortality—less than 1 to 5 percent
Neurologic complication—less than 1 to 5 percent
Infection—0.5 to 5 percent

Chapter 7

Denying Your Scoliosis and Refusing Treatment

Many people slip into the comfort zone of denial when faced with a diagnosis of scoliosis. Others employ this technique when surgical needs escalate and action is needed. But delaying effective coping and decision-making related to your scoliosis may be setting the stage for more drastic measures at a later date.

There are a multitude of reasons why someone would use avoidance. Some people are obstinate toward doctors, too easily convinced by promises of correction with alternative treatments, afraid of surgery or needles, uneducated about scoliosis, or just not ready to acknowledge it—and this is not effective coping. While complications from surgery are a concern, you need to know that neglecting a curve that is becoming progressively worse makes the prospect of surgery that much more difficult and dangerous.

THE LACK OF MONEY OR INSURANCE PREVENTING TREATMENT

If money or lack of insurance coverage is a problem, Shriners' is always a viable option for children. Also, you can talk to the billing department at your hospital for possible payment options that can be broken up incrementally over time. You can seek advice from your surgeon or HMO, too.

OLDER ADULTS WHO ARE NOT SURGICAL CANDIDATES

There comes a point in life when the dangers associated with surgery outweigh the benefits, and when having corrective surgery would cause you more pain and difficulty—*unnecessary* pain and difficulty—than not having surgery.

ALTERNATIVE TREATMENTS

Recently I sought treatment from a local chiropractor because I had been rehearsing feverishly for an upcoming ballet and was experiencing a fair amount of back discomfort. So, three times a week I visited my chiropractor, where I received electrical stimulation treatments. Unaware of my knowledge in the field of scoliosis and my role as president of the Scoliosis Association of Connecticut, this chiropractor was very encouraging about the success of my treatments. Success to me meant pain relief and, indeed, my pain was being relieved. There was never much conversation during my treatments and certainly, clarification of the word "success" never occurred to me. After several weeks of treatment, my mother came to one of my appointments. The chiropractor was very excited and said that he felt that by Christmas he would have a surprise for us. My mother asked, "What is it?" He said, "I think we might be able to prevent Brooke from having scoliosis surgery!" My mother and I just looked at him with surprise, smiled, and left the office.

While there *are* many alternative pain management treatments, there are very few alternative treatments for preventing the progression of scoliosis and *none* for correcting scoliosis.

ERIC
"Searching for an Alternative to Surgery"
Eric had been checked by his pediatrician as a child and found to have a slight curvature. His parents took him to an orthopedic surgeon, who assured them there was nothing to worry about. Soon, however, Eric's

parents began to notice a marked protrusion of his right scapula, which they referred to as the "hump becoming more prominent." They went back to their pediatrician to once again have him checked, and the pediatrician responded by saying, "Oh, this is the scoliosis we talked about." This was the first time they heard the word "scoliosis." In the winter of 1996, Eric once again visited an orthopedic surgeon, where he was X-rayed and diagnosed as having a thoracic curve of forty to forty-two degrees. This came as a surprise to the family, because there was no known history of scoliosis in the family. Subsequently, however, his sister, age fourteen, was diagnosed with a twelve-degree curve. His older brother remains scoliosis free. At the time, Eric was

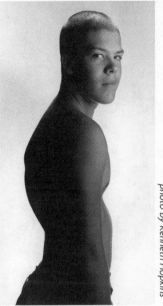

photo by Kenneth Hopkins

fifteen and not a candidate for bracing. Surgery was the recommended mode of treatment. The family sought a second opinion, which concurred with the first.

At this point the family was not ready to face Eric having surgery. They decided to seek an alternative to surgery and did so by spending much time researching scoliosis on the Internet. They found a chiropractor in Wisconsin who claimed to correct scoliosis. Eric and his dad flew out to Wisconsin to meet this man. They brought the protocol back to Connecticut and searched for a local chiropractor who had the necessary table and equipment and the willingness to implement the prescribed exercise regime. They located a chiropractor who agreed to try this program, but who was also quite uncertain about the outcome.

The prescribed program consisted of a visit to the chiropractor's office three times per week for a treatment on a flexion table, with pressure applied for certain periods of time. In addition, a bar was installed in his room at home from which he was to hang two times per day, for two minutes each time. Then Eric progressed to pullups. The treatment also suggested that he use free weights, bench pressing, and breathing exercises twice a day. Eric embarked upon this regime for a total of four months before the next set of X rays were taken.

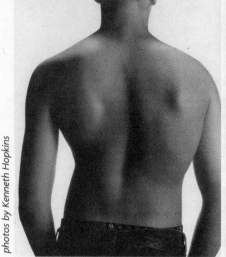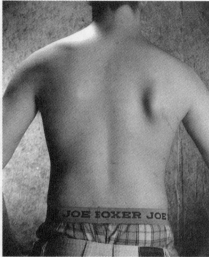

photos by Kenneth Hopkins

*Left: Eric before surgery. **Right:** Eric After surgery.*

In the fall of 1997, after four months, Eric and his family traveled to New York City to visit a chiropractor who had the machine necessary to take "hanging X rays" which, they were told, "gave a more accurate reading." Eric's scoliosis had progressed. By the following January, Eric's family and the local chiropractor agreed that the treatment was, in fact, not working, and that surgery was in order.

Eric's dad got on the Internet every day and posted questions regarding "alternative surgery." A doctor from California responded by explaining the newest procedure for thoracic correction called an Anterior Spinal Fusion, using a thoracoscopic approach (see chapter 5). He was put in touch with a nearby doctor who would perform this operation.

Spring brought a journey to Philadelphia's Shriners' Hospital, where Eric satisfied the criteria and was found to be a "perfect" candidate for this type of surgery. The benefit of this type of approach through port-holes is less instrumentation because the rods are smaller and less scarring. They were told the surgery would take approximately eight hours and that during this surgery, Eric's right lung would be deflated to prevent puncturing. He journeyed to Shriners' two weeks before the surgery to undergo pulmonary function tests, nerve conduction study, and to donate blood. He would be allowed to stay at the hospital for a week to ten days because it was a Shriners' hospital, where insurance does not dictate the length of stay.

On August 23, 1998, Eric entered surgery with a curve in the seventy-degree range and had his scoliosis corrected with what ended up being a modified version of a thoracoscopic approach. When they deflated his right lung, his oxygen level decreased significantly because the left lung wasn't supplying him with enough oxygen. The doctors reinflated the right lung and tried again. After two unsuccessful attempts, the doctors inflated his lung and ended up connecting the portals and making an anterior incision, which had a successful fusion of levels T5 to T12. The surgery took nine hours; Eric's seventy-degree curve was corrected to approximately forty degrees. He remained at Shriners' for ten days before journeying home to Connecticut. His hospital stay was "fabulous!" His parents were housed at a nearby Ronald McDonald House which cost fifteen dollars a night for the first three nights, then ten dollars a night thereafter.

DAVID
"I Never Go Anywhere without My Basketball."

David is an eighty-three-year-old retired optometrist who is five feet, three inches tall. He was diagnosed at age seven with scoliosis, but never allowed it to hamper the things he loved to do.

He had surgery as a teenager for a right thoracic curve—over sixty-five years ago. He remembers being hospitalized for a period of two

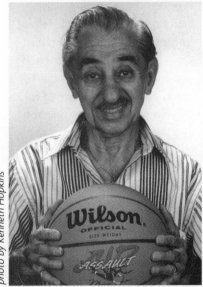

photo by Kenneth Hopkins

months and wore a plaster cast for many months after that. Upon removal of the cast, he was put into a brace until his teenage years were over. David inherited his scoliosis from his dad. Naturally, he was concerned about this hereditary trait when he married. Fortunately, his children—now ages fifty and fifty-three—do not have scoliosis. And neither do his grandchildren!

To this day, David maintains that he is pain-free. His back deformity is visible, and he lives with asymmetry in leg and arm lengths. However, to know and see this gentleman brings joy to one's day. David has been active in sports since the age of ten—basketball is his favorite! By the age of sixty-nine, he had glided through several Senior Olympic competitions, amassing a grand total of forty-seven awards in a three-and-a-half-year period; he won a gold medal in basketball and a bronze in bocci ball, and captured ten medals in the U.S. Senior Athletic Games. Today, David competes in various senior citizen Olympics throughout Florida. He never goes anywhere without his basketball, which stays in the back of his car. As a matter of fact, David was bouncing the ball around during my interview with him!

SYLVIA

"I Had More Discomfort in My Forties than I Have Today, in My Eighties!"

To look at Sylvia, one would never suspect that she is eighty-five years old. A petite blonde, impeccably dressed and manicured, Sylvia has lived with scoliosis since the age of eleven. Sylvia inherited her scoliosis from her mother and had a brother two years her senior who also had scoliosis. While her brother wore a brace for two years, bracing was not for her; she refused to wear the brace when scoliosis was diagnosed by the clinic. As an alternative, she was given exercises to do, which she still does today. Her love for theater in her teens and twenties led her to join a theater group, and she remained active in theater until just ten years ago.

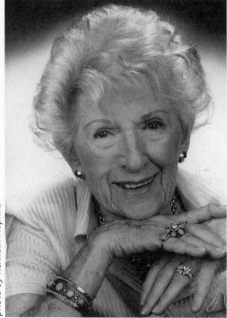

photo by Kenneth Hopkins

When Sylvia went off to college, she began figure skating, learned to dance at Rockefeller Center, and began to paint. Only painting caused her back discomfort. She went on to marry and has been married for fifty-six years; she has one son and three grandchildren.

Today, her posture is beautiful, although she does have a very visible right thoracic hump. She has one leg longer than the other, which yields uneven hips; however, this disfigurement is camouflaged by her stunning appearance and beautiful smile. She exercises religiously every day and has had to increase her exercises over the years to treat her sciatica and arthritis. Her daily regime consists of floor exercises, weightlifting, and forty jumping jacks.

CHARLIE
"Living with a 125 Degree Curve"

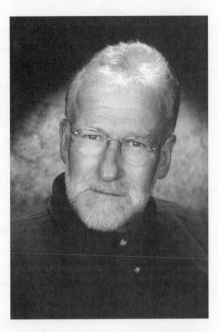

At age fifty, Charlie revealed to me his lifelong battle with scoliosis for the first time. With no family history whatsoever, Charlie, one of five children, was diagnosed at age two with congenital scoliosis during a routine pediatric visit. His parents were told by the physician that there was an operation available, but recommended that he just be watched.

And so, life went on, no one ever spoke about it, and scoliosis became the "family secret." Charlie's mother's greatest fear was that if his scoliosis were "fixed," he would be sent to Vietnam. As Charlie grew older, he was not allowed to play any sports for fear that he would hurt his back. His family encouraged him to keep himself covered up. "Tell people you burn easily when you're at the beach," they would say.

In college, he tried skiing but his doctor discouraged it. He did, however, play full contact sports as a hobby. While he remained asymptomatic, the pain he experienced was in his heart. He was taunted by kids about his obvious deformity. He fought back in his own way by taking up fighting and boxing as

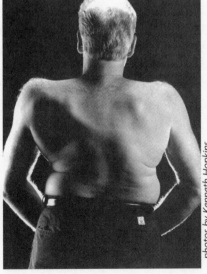

photos by Kenneth Hopkins

hobbies in which he excelled because of his very long arm span (typical in scoliosis patients). Still, it was difficult for Charlie to cope. Everyone in his family was tall—at least six-foot-four; Charlie grew to five feet, ten inches. This bothered him, so the family sought the help of a psychiatrist.

Along the way, Charlie was followed closely by orthopedic doctors who kept a close watch on him with X rays. Often, he remembers the appointments as full-day events. In 1972, at age twenty-five, his orthopedic surgeon was not very encouraging and referred him to Dr. Harrington, the scoliosis surgeon who invented the Harrington Rod. Charlie contemplated surgery at this time, but decided against it. Again, at age thirty, he sought the advice of yet another scoliosis surgeon who, at this point, highly recommended surgery, pointing out what the future might hold for him if he declined surgery. Charlie did not elect to have surgery because, he said, it would have been impossible for him to take a year off; he was married and about to start a family. In the early 1980s, his X rays revealed a thoracic curve of 110 to 115 degrees. But, this time, the doctor told him his spine was fused and surgery was not recommended. In the mid-1980s, he sprained his back. Again, the doctor simply prescribed muscle relaxants and never mentioned the word surgery.

Today, Charlie has a successful career as a licensed professional engineer. He is happily married with three beautiful children. His daughter was thought to have scoliosis at about six months. But, by eighteen months to two years, any trace of it had vanished. His two sons stand tall at six feet, two inches and six feet, three inches. Charlie keeps in shape by doing situps—he has an incredibly strong abdomen—and he walks on the treadmill at 4.2 miles per hour for 45 minutes each day. He is observed regularly by a cardiologist and a pulmonologist. While Charlie does have decreased lung capacity, he remains asymptomatic with the exception of occasional shooting pains down his limbs. Charlie is living successfully with an untreated scoliosis, which now measures 125 degrees and he stands very tall at five feet, eight inches. His greatest regret is not talking about scoliosis more openly—to this day, he keeps covered up at the beach. I thank Charlie, a very private man, for opening up and sharing his story in hopes of helping others.

Chapter 8

Pain Management Techniques for Scoliosis Patients

While the incidence of back pain in scoliosis approximates that of the general population (sixty to ninety percent), the severity of the pain in scoliosis patients tends to be greater. There can be several causes of scoliotic pain. One might be muscle fatigue and soreness caused by the muscles' constant effort at posture correction and compensation. Pain may result from joint inflammation and degeneration in the curving spine. Arthritic degeneration can be a contributor. Radicular pain can be generated by nerve compression. In large curves, the ribs may press together. While surgery may be considered in part to alleviate pain, that intervention itself has its own sources of discomfort.

The pain from scoliosis can have a wide range of intensity, from none through acute and chronic pain. Since most people with scoliosis will experience at least discomfort at some time in their lives, let's take a closer look at the subject of pain with an eye toward pain treatment and management.

WHAT IS PAIN?

In general, pain is a part of our body's self-protection and survival system. It is a signal that tells us that something is wrong and a message that urges our attention.

POTENTIAL DISCOMFORT RANGE AND EXAMPLES			
Severity:	None	Discomfort	Acute	Chronic/Over Time
Possible Sources:		bracing	surgery muscle spasms pinched nerve	muscle fatigue multiple surgeries arthritic degeneration other conditions secondary to lifelong scoliosis

ACUTE PAIN

Physiologically, when a part of our body is damaged or hurt, the nerves in that area are stimulated. The nerve endings, or *pain receptors*, react to damage and transmit the information from one bundle of nerve fibers to another. These nerve fibers are channeled through the spinal cord and up to the brain. This is called the *ascending tract*. The chemical substances in each nerve of the tract, which actually carry the signal to the brain, are called *neurotransmitters*. When this signal is perceived, interpreted, and evaluated by the brain along several different pathways involving emotions and thoughts, we experience pain.

It is important to note that there is not a one-to-one correspondence between a pain signal and our subjective experience of and reaction to pain. Consider the situation of an injured athlete or a severely wounded soldier who continues to perform despite serious bodily damage. In these situations, the persons involved often report reduced awareness of their pain until they have finished their required tasks. Their brains and bodies respond to their injuries with natural neurotransmitter painkillers called *endorphins*. As such, our brains produce chemical responses along the *descending tract* in nerve transmission. This can actually diminish the pain signal. Indeed, there is a continuously interacting feedback loop between pain signals and brain responses to those signals, between the ascending and descending tracts. In short, brain activity can influence and reduce pain sensation.

CHRONIC PAIN

When acute pain gets the attention it needs or the damage heals, the pain generally subsides. However, when pain persists over time, say for more than six months, the condition is known as chronic pain. When pain continues or reoccurs over weeks, months, and even years, most people report feeling anxious, fearful, hopeless, and depressed. They see no end to their suffering and no light at the end of the tunnel. The more depressed they feel, the more vulnerable they are to the pain experienced. Anger, hostility, and frustration can become daily emotional states. Disturbed family relationships, problems at work, conflicts with doctors, and increased alcohol and substance abuse become ongoing life themes. For chronic pain patients, the pain itself is as central a problem as any scoliosis factor from which it might arise.

FACTORS INFLUENCING PAIN EXPERIENCES

Chronic pain involves nearly all of a person's physical, psychological, and social systems. A number of factors all act together to influence the pain experience. They can alter our threshold for the experience of pain.

◆ *Activity level:* What do I do when I experience pain? Do I tense up or remain relaxed? Am I active or passive? Do I know what to do at those times? Activity can directly influence our thoughts and emotions.

◆ *Emotional states:* How do I feel during pain? Examples might be fearful, helpless, or angry.

◆ *Sensory factors:* Where do I feel pain? How intense is the pain? What is the quality of the pain (dull or burning vs. sharp and stabbing)? At what times do I feel the pain? When is it lessened?

◆ *Cognitive factors:* What thoughts accompany pain sensations (*e.g.*, "I can't handle this" vs. "I know this will pass")? What images go through my mind (*e.g.*, "This pain is like a hot knife on my back" vs. "I feel the pressure on my back")? Thoughts and images determine the focus of our attention.

◆ *Social factors:* How do family and friends, health professionals, employers and co-workers react to my pain? How do I interact with them? What do I talk about when I am with them?

◆ *Biological/medication/analgesic factors:* What medications help me during pain episodes? Do I use them appropriately? Is there a working partnership among myself, my physician/pain specialist, and my pharmacist so that I am following a regimen that's best for me? Am I doing physical therapy?

These six areas form the foundation of what is called a biopsychosocial approach to pain treatment and management. Given the constant interaction between brain and pain or mind and body, biology/physiology, psychology, and social factors all interact to either lower or raise a person's threshold for pain awareness. The higher the threshold, the lower is the self-report of pain.

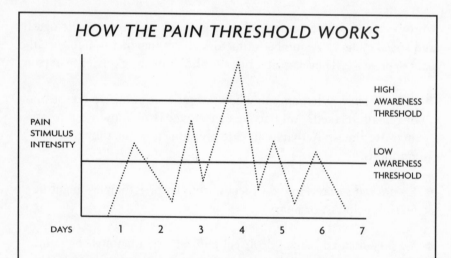

HOW THE PAIN THRESHOLD WORKS

PAIN STIMULUS INTENSITY

HIGH AWARENESS THRESHOLD

LOW AWARENESS THRESHOLD

DAYS   1   2   3   4   5   6   7

As can be seen in this example, although pain stimulus may fluctuate from day to day, the pain threshold determines a person's awareness of and reaction to that stimulus. This hypothetical individual had five significant pain events. However, the high threshold state would produce only one pain awareness experience. The low threshold state would result in an experience of all five events. Clearly, the goal is to raise one's threshold to the experience of pain.

A BIOPSYCHOSOCIAL APPROACH TO PAIN TREATMENT AND MANAGEMENT

A biopsychosocial approach to the self-management of pain works with all of the preceding factors that influence pain. As such, this approach gives the person a wide range of strategies and methods to use when managing pain on a daily basis. Remember, each factor interacts with other factors—for example, how we *think* and what we *do* about pain can influence our *feelings* and *images* about pain, which, in turn, can alter our pain *sensation*. As such, the more strategies we use, the better our chances for altering or even blocking pain signals.

Fortunately, in our society today, we have a variety of both traditional medical as well as alternative methods of pain management from which to choose. Although each method has validity, there is no "best" or "only" way of managing pain. Often people find that several techniques or methods work best when used in conjunction with another. Some persons combine both medical as well as nonmedical approaches for best relief. Find out what works best for you. Setting realistic goals, eliciting the support of others, and helping yourself is as an important part of pain management as the techniques themselves. All of these things will help you to work against the feeling that you are a victim of your pain.

When using medical, nonmedical, or a combination of approaches to help manage your pain, a good rule of thumb is to try and find a doctor, practitioner, or instructor who has had experience in working with people who have scoliosis pain. Find out not only the pros, but also the possible cons in using a particular method. Are there side effects, does this method suit you emotionally and physically, and can you set realistic goals? Talk to your medical professional about your concerns and expectations. Do your own research by reading current material, checking things out with an established support network, or by using the Internet.

BIOLOGICAL / MEDICAL APPROACHES

MEDICATION

There are many types of medicines used for the control of pain. However, some medications that are beneficial for handling acute pain may not be sufficient for the treatment of chronic pain. Other medications may actually complicate matters with unpleasant side effects. This is particularly true of narcotic analgesics, minor tranquilizers, and sedatives. As such, use medications as prescribed by your physician, your surgeon, or your psychiatrist. Your pain level, physical condition, age, and other factors will be taken into account, and you will be able to "fine tune" a regimen that addresses your needs.

The following are categories of medicines used in pain treatment and management and some of the more common and familiar examples:

Narcotic Analgesics
Morphine
Codeine
Hydromorphine (Dilaudid)
Percocet
Demerol

Non-Steroidal Anti-Inflammatory Drugs (NSAIDs)
Aspirin
Ibuprofen
Naproxen
Indomethacin

Major Tranquilizers
Haldol
Mellaril
Navane
Proloxin

Non-Narcotic Analgesics
Acetaminophen (Tylenol)
Darvocet or Darvon
Vicodin (Hydrocodone)

Antidepressants
Amitriptyline (Elavil)
Selective Serotonin Reuptake Inhibitors (SSRIs):
    Prozac
    Zoloft
Effexor
Wellbutrin

Minor Tranquilizers
Valium
Xanax
Ativan

Other
Neurontin

Pain management is a complex subject and takes into account several factors, including the type of scoliosis, the type of surgery that is performed, the patient's age, psychological status, motivation, and tissue response to surgical trauma. The post-surgical patient presents the most challenge in terms of medication usage. For most adolescents and young patients undergoing spinal surgery, the initial use of narcotic medications given intravenously or intramuscularly is usually replaced with oral analgesics (painkillers) shortly after surgery. Most patients are discharged within five to seven days with oral analgesics, which could be either Percocet, Vicodin, Tylenol III, Darvocet, or a similar analgesic. Most adolescents and young patients are usually free of narcotic medication use in two to three weeks, and within a month do not require any stronger medication than plain Tylenol. Anti-inflammatory medications are usually not recommended for the sake of possible interference with the fusion of the spine.

On the other hand, adults tend to have more complex medication and pain issues post-operatively. Besides the use of stronger narcotics intravenously in the immediate post-operative period, adults may require the help of a chronic pain management program thereafter, which could extend into weeks and, in some cases, months. This will require a multidisciplinary approach to pain management, including seeing pain consultants such as anesthesiologists and also psychologists and psychiatrists. Medications range from morphine, Dilaudid, Percocet, and Duragesic patches; these are usually used singularly or in combination, and must be closely monitored by a single physician who also has close ties with the patient. Patients are monitored during the chronic pain management program and are weaned off these medications on an individual basis. However, there are some patients who, despite doctors' aggressive measures to wean them from the medication, still require pain medicine for the sake of continuing pain. Such chronic pain syndromes, despite a stable, solid fusion in some patients with complex issues, are best treated by a chronic pain expert.

A Word about Antidepressants and Pain Management. As said before, there is a close connection between chronic pain and depression. Most people with chronic pain report symptoms of depression: low energy, feeling helpless and hopeless, changes in appetite, disturbed sleep, and feelings of sadness. Many people with depression also have pain complaints. The common link between pain and depression is the neurotransmitter called serotonin. Chronic pain lowers the amount of serotonin in the brain, thereby causing depression and lowering the threshold of pain. Depressed people are more vulnerable to pain.

Many of the new antidepressants (especially the SSRI category) work directly to increase serotonin levels. In doing so, they raise the pain threshold. Many people who take antidepressants report considerable relief from their discomfort. In many cases, the dosage of antidepressant is lower than the dose used when treating significant, clinical depression. If you experience long-term pain, discuss the possible use of antidepressants with your doctor. He or she will know your medical condition, will be aware of any contraindications, and will inform you of any possible side effects you will encounter. Antidepressants can make a significant difference in your daily life and activities!

RELAXATION TECHNIQUES

Relaxation techniques are especially important to learn when coping with pain. They are particularly useful in countering the tension and stress that can accompany pain, thereby magnifying its intensity. Since we cannot be tense and relaxed at the same time, these techniques go right to the heart of pain control.

Regular Abdominal Breathing. People who are relaxed breathe more slowly and deeply from their abdomens. Practice abdominal (diaphragmatic) breathing. Inhale slowly and deeply through your nose into the "bottom" of your lungs, as low as you can go. Your abdomen should actually rise slightly. Pause for a count of four or five, and exhale slowly through your mouth. As you exhale, allow your body to just let go. You might visualize your arms and legs going loose and limp like a rag doll's. Each time you exhale, think the word "calm" or "relax" or "serene." Do several full abdominal breaths. Keep your breathing smooth and regular. This will result in increased oxygen supply to the brain and muscles, thus promoting a feeling of calmness and quiescence.

Progressive Muscle Relaxation. Systematically tense (for seven to ten seconds) and then relax the various muscle groups of the body. Proceed from your hands, arms, and face to your shoulders, chest, abdomen, legs, and feet. The entire process should take you about twenty minutes. With practice, you should be able to relax your body just by focusing on, or thinking about, the various muscle groups in succession.

Visualization and Meditation. After completing progressive muscle relaxation, it is helpful to visualize yourself in the midst of a peaceful scene. This will help free you from anxious thoughts and distract you from your pain. The scene can be a quiet beach, a mountain lake, or any calming place (where you are safe and alone). Picture all the details of the scene, and involve yourself completely with each of your five senses. What do you see, hear, smell, feel, and sense? You don't need to restrict yourself to reality—imagining yourself floating on a cloud is just as effective. The point here is to absorb yourself completely in the mental picture, with all of your attention. Focus only on one thing at a time to counteract distraction.

In a similar manner, meditation—the letting go of thoughts about the immediate past or future, and just simply "being" in the present—can be quite effective in reducing stress and tension caused by pain. Meditation has been with us for about five thousand years, and many texts have been written about its various forms. Because it has withstood the test of time, many pain specialists recommend meditation as part of a comprehensive pain management program. It is interesting to note that the principles of visualization and meditation are also used in the highly effective modality of self hypnosis for pain management.

Biofeedback. Biofeedback monitors heart rate, blood pressure, skin temperature, and muscle tension. It can help you to learn how you feel when your muscles are tense or relaxed so you can learn to control your body's responses to pain. Biofeedback has helped many scoliosis patients to avoid undue pain and suffering, assisting them in getting back on their feet and in control of their destinies. Biofeedback is not a panacea; it is just one of the best tools available for minimizing pain. But what, exactly, is this *thing* known as biofeedback?

Biofeedback helps to monitor the progress of relaxation by giving information or "feedback" about the levels of stress and tension in the body. Electrodes are attached to various muscle groups. When muscles are tense, their electrical output increases. The electrodes measure the output, and the results are displayed on a television monitor and/or by a tone that beeps faster and louder with increased tension, slower and softer with decreased tension. Biofeedback can also measure heart rate, amout of sweat produced, temperature, and blood pressure. Through biofeedback, people learn the often subtle body cues associated with stressed and relaxed physiological states. They can learn to better control painful muscle spasms, as well as clenching, tension, and contraction often associated with pain episodes.

Using biofeedback can help you to regain your muscle function or to control your blood pressure following scoliosis surgery; it can also help you to take control of your body and to manage pain if you have not had surgery. Ask your doctor about biofeedback and what it can do for you. Those who have tried it seem to have nothing but praise for the treatment.

Music Therapy. Music therapy is the use of music as a method of treatment, one that brings about a change from an unhealthy or painful situation to a healthy or more pleasurable state. What makes it such a useful tool is that each of us can relate to and respond to the universal nonverbal language of music. Indeed, music can and does influence human behavior and, as with imagery, music can effect powerful emotional and physiological changes in us.

Music therapy is often used in conjunction with other modalities for pain management, such as relaxation and visualization. Sometimes people have difficulty relaxing their body or mind and directing their thoughts or images in a way that lessens their pain response. In these cases, music can help to relax your body and guide your imagery.

If you are having pain and are sensitive to lights, sounds, and other distractions in the environment, you may not be able to relax your body enough to focus your thoughts. Sometimes listening to a quiet, relaxing piece of music helps to progressively bring your body into a more relaxed state and guide your thoughts. Using the same methods of relaxation and visualization previously discussed, the overall therapeutic result using music can be even more effective because music helps bypass pain centers in the brain.

For example, let's say you are scheduled for scoliosis surgery. Six to eight weeks before your surgery, begin to practice progressive relaxation and guided imagery with music. You need to practice consistently to achieve an effective relaxation response. You may find that eventually, just by turning on a particular piece of music, your body will have an automatic conditioned relaxation response without your having to work at it. Your mind associates the music with a pleasurable, relaxed state and produces an automatic physiological response.

This method can be especially helpful for presurgical anxiety and for any pain you may have in the several weeks after the surgery. If you have difficulty with this method even after practicing, make an appointment with a therapist who can coach you for a few sessions.

Chiropractic. Some people prefer to go to a chiropractor for treatment of their scoliosis and/or pain. Chiropractors manipulate the spine to correct subluxations or misalignment of the vertebrae. A qualified doctor of chiropractic can suggest a treatment plan for you, depending on your age and the type of scoliosis you have. Many people have curves that remain small and never progress. Some curves, especially in growing prepubescent children, have a history of rapid progression. If, during the course of your chiropractic treatment, your curve increases, you may opt to discontinue treatment with your chiropractor for pain. However, get an evaluation with an orthopedist for your curve.

Physiatry. Physiatrists are medical doctors who specialize in physical medicine and rehabilitation. Many work in conjunction with physical therapists. If you have scoliosis and wear a brace, have surgery, or have intermittent or chronic pain, a consultation with a physiatrist can be invaluable. Physiatrists make use of a variety of nonsurgical techniques to decrease pain, strengthen muscles, and improve the quality of life. Pain management clinics often have a physiatrist on staff.

Massage. Therapeutic massage is a wonderful pain management modality. It's hard to imagine a better way to deal with muscle strain and fatigue, spasms, or any physical discomfort or pain experienced with scoliosis. Massage is also an excellent pain reliever for secondary problems related to scoliosis that may occur as one ages; for example, sciatica and arthritis. About the only contraindication for massage in relation to scoliosis would be inflammatory disc problems.

Some of the goals in using massage for scoliosis would be to stretch tightened structures, strengthen weak muscles, and improve ventilation and mobility. The therapist accomplishes this by using passive exercises and specific massage strokes to bring nutrition to the muscles and to relieve pain. The massage therapist will sometimes hold the back muscles in symmetrical and carefully corrected positions that help to re-educate muscle sense as well as strengthen muscles.

Make sure the therapist you choose is licensed. Most states require 500-plus hours of classroom training, and some, an additional state board exam to become a licensed massage therapist. Although massage therapists study pathology, it is best to find a therapist who has worked with scoliosis clients. You can start by asking for a referral from your medical doctor or chiropractor. You may have to evaluate a few massage therapists until you find someone who has a technique with which you feel comfortable.

For those individuals who have had surgery and who now have

hardware, you will probably feel more comfortable with massage once pain and swelling have lessened. Make sure that your therapist knows you have hardware, as well as any other medical conditions. That way, your massage can be tailored to your individual needs.

Heat and Cold Treatments. Heat and cold therapy help reduce pain, stiffness, and spasm. Generally speaking, cold packs can numb the affected area and are more important in the treatment of muscle injury and inflammation. Heat treatment can relax the muscles. Dry heat methods most commonly used are heating pads and heat lamps. Moist heat methods include a warm bath or shower or hydrocolator packs. If you have hardware, follow the advice of your doctor or physical therapist when using these methods. This is especially important for people who have hardware!

PSYCHOLOGICAL FACTORS

How we think has a direct impact on how we feel. When it comes to the management of pain, negative thinking can actually increase anxiety, stress, depression, and pain. As such, it is most important to discover any patterns of negative thinking that we might have and to replace them with healthier, positive, more adaptive modes of thought.

NEGATIVE THINKING STYLES

Negative thinking styles form the basis of negative self-statements and, as such, of negative emotions and feeling states. They can take a perfectly neutral event in our lives, distort it, and then make us feel negatively toward it. Imagine what they can do to a less than positive event like pain! Let's look at some of these distorted thinking styles and the negative statements and feeling states they might generate.

Catastrophizing. This style of thinking automatically assumes the worst possible outcome. It is characterized by "what if" statements. For example, "What if this pain will never go away?" or "What if I can't cope this time?" It locks us out of positive outcomes and solutions, thereby diminishing hope. It can escalate any worries we can have about an already problematic situation.

Shoulds. Shoulds are the foundation of distorted thinking. Statements with words like "should," "ought," and "must" fit into this distortion. Some common examples might be, "I *should* not have this pain," or "I *should* never have scoliosis," or "I *ought to* be perfect," or "I *must* have done something to bring this on." These and many more statements can set standards that are inflexible, life-restricting, and unrealistic. With "should" statements, we often blame ourselves for the very situation we would like to avoid.

Overgeneralization. With this distortion, we come to a general conclusion based on a single incident or piece of evidence. Key distortion words are "never," "always," "all," "every," "none," and "nobody." For example, "I'll *never* get over this," or "*Nobody* cares about my pain," or "Will I *always* feel like this?" or "I feel pain. This program will *never* work."

Emotional Reasoning. With this error, we automatically assume that what we feel must be true. "I feel afraid that this pain won't stop" equals "This pain won't stop." Or, "I'm worried that I won't get back to work" equals "I won't ever work again." Or, "I feel worthless" equals "I am worthless." The reality is that the world looks better when the intense emotions settle down.

These styles of thinking can all interact to weave a negative fabric of self-statements in response to pain: "Here comes that spasm again. I won't be able to work tomorrow. I know the pain medications can't handle this. This will wipe me out. This body of mine is good for nothing." Such an internal monologue can result in anxiety, panic, depression, and self-deprecation. It can actually shut us out of effective strategies for coping with pain and actually magnify one's awareness of the pain itself.

HOW TO COMBAT DISTORTED THINKING

◆ *Analyze your thoughts.* Many thoughts come quickly and almost automatically. You must carefully monitor yourself to see which negative thinking styles you are apt to use and identify these styles before you can correct them.

◆ *Recognize the negative emotions you have as a result of using the distorted thinking styles.* Most of us are locked into emotional response patterns based on the thoughts we have. Feeling anxious, angry, or depressed can be cues that you are using a particular distortion; negative feelings are the consequences of negative beliefs.

◆ *Develop a set of coping statements based on positive, reasonable considerations.* You might write positive coping statements down and keep them with you. Some examples might be:
- This pain will pass. It always has.
- Don't jump to conclusions just because you're anxious.
- I know how to cope with this. I've done it before.
- Just breathe deeply. Release that tension in my shoulders.
- Don't expect the worst. Time may bring relief.

◆ *Talk yourself through the pain episode.* Use your coping statements. Use other effective strategies to keep yourself in control.

Psychological approaches to pain management can be highly effective, especially when used in conjunction with the biological/medical approaches previously discussed. Together, they form two-thirds of a multidimensional pain control strategy. Let's look at the third part of the plan.

SOCIAL APPROACHES

Social approaches are concerned with effective interpersonal activity. These approaches are important since people with chronic pain are not always in their emotional best form.

ASSERTIVENESS

Many people who cope with ongoing pain find that their emotions shift from depression to anger. When feeling down, many such people find little energy for interpersonal activities such as conversations, phone calls, or letter writing. In this depressed mode, a person may not get his or her needs met and is often not up to talking with others who might be of help and assistance. Over time, this can result in fewer contacts with friends, relations, and others. A passive, isolated lifestyle can be an unfortunate consequence.

When in an angry mode, many individuals in pain are too confrontational and hostile in interpersonal endeavors, which results in ineffective interpersonal outcomes and often unmet needs. Angry individuals can "turn off" the very professionals and others on whom they need to depend. Doctors, spouse, family members, and friends will tend to withdraw from the hostile pain patient. Again, isolation is the result.

Furthermore, people who are unassertive in their behavior often do not believe that they have a right to their feelings, opinions, or concerns. They do not stand up for themselves. They do not feel what others tell them. Consequently, they become generally frustrated.

The following are guidelines that promote assertive, effective, interpersonal behavior. They are especially important to remember when feeling angry or depressed.

- Assertion is not the same as aggression. Say and do just what the situation requires—no more, no less.
- Maintain good eye contact. Avoid staring.
- Remember to be friendly. Smile appropriately.
- Speak clearly and loudly enough to be heard. Identify what it is you want or need; be clear about what you don't want or don't need.
- Be respectful. Avoid sarcasm and ridicule. Avoid overly apologetic behavior. Avoid power gestures like finger pointing or clenching a fist.
- Don't ramble on. When you've stated what it is you wanted, or when you've made your point, stop talking.
- Remember to listen. Ask for clarifications when needed.

Appropriate assertion can go a long way toward getting your needs met. It can made you feel effective when you may not be up to the task.

PROBLEM SOLVING SKILLS

Individuals with pain often report that they are not thinking clearly about effective solutions to their problems. As a consequence, they sometimes choose solutions that are ineffective and counterproductive. Many depressed people say they can't cope. What they really mean is that they can't define their problem nor find a reasonable solution to it. The following are suggestions for more effective problem solving.

- State the problem clearly. It often helps to write the problem out first before talking about it. The use of words puts boundaries on vague and unclear issues, and writing about the problem can help you to face the issues directly.
- Avoid negative thinking.
- Brainstorm all possible solutions to the problem, even odd or silly ones. Write them out.
- List all the pros and cons of each brainstorm item.
- Rank your solutions in the order of best to worst.
- Define time limits for acting on a solution.
- Congratulate yourself for solving the problem!

PUTTING IT ALL TOGETHER

The biopsychosocial approach to pain management provides a wide array of strategies to pain treatment and control. Here is an example of thoughts and actions that might be used to raise the pain threshold when coping with a pain episode:

- Stop and ask, "Can I can learn anything from this pain episode? Is there a trigger I might not have realized before? Have I followed the physical therapy regimen?"
- Use slow abdominal breathing. Calm myself.
- Ask, "What are my alternatives in approaching this episode?"
- What distracting activities can I engage in? Can I watch television or rent a movie?
- Is medicine appropriate?
- Should I use cold compresses? Should I take a hot shower?

- Can I do visualization or other relaxation exercises? Can I do self-hypnosis?
- Engage in positive, coping thoughts such as, "I know how to cope. I've been here before. This will pass." Calm myself.
- Can I talk with anyone to distract myself? Can I plan my next vacation? Can I go on-line?

The more techniques you employ, the higher your threshold for pain experience will be.

CHAPTER 9

How to Cope with Physical Challenges and Stigma on a Daily Basis

What makes one person with a severe physical injury (*e.g.*, an amputated limb) become isolated, angry, and depressed while another person with the same condition remains self-assured, socially active, and even enters athletic competitions? Recent research is uncovering three findings to answer such a question:

1. How we *perceive* stigma can negatively affect our self-esteem and can increase depression.
2. The more social support we have, the greater our sense of self-worth.
3. The fewer the number of daily life hassles and negative life events we experience, the better is the level of adjustment and the fewer the number of self-reported symptoms.

Let's take a closer look at these factors in terms of scoliosis.

PERCEIVED STIGMA

The concept of perceived stigma refers to how a person sees or understands her scoliosis condition as *part* of herself and not her *entire* self.

It also refers to how a person with scoliosis thinks that *other people* notice his curve or will respond to him as deformed, disabled, or physically limited. Ultimately, we must conquer stigma from within ourselves. Here are some directions to consider when combating stigma:

◆ Make sure you *accurately* perceive your physical situation. Many people look at their curve or surgical scar and believe that the curve or scar totally defines them. They are using a *part* of themselves to define the *whole* of themselves. Avoid "part" perceptions. Look at the whole of you, not just one aspect of you. This is a first step toward balanced self-perception.

◆ Look at your strengths and assets, not simply your limitations. People who look only at limitations fail to get the big picture. They distort themselves and label their actual achievements as shortcomings (*e.g.*, "I only got a 95 on that school exam. Why didn't I get 100? What a dunce I am."). Remember that the world may actually perceive your "limitations" as strengths (*e.g.*, a scar as a badge of courage vs. a scar as a deformity), so why don't you? You have enough to deal with. Be a friend to yourself. See yourself as others see you. Be aware of your strengths, achievements, skills, successes, and accomplishments. Regularly remind yourself about them.

◆ Remember that how you view yourself directly affects how others view you. In other words, the confidence and self-assurance you project will determine how others react to you and to your scoliosis. The previous two factors (accurate self-perception and awareness of strengths) can directly raise your self-confidence and self-esteem. They will be evident in your self-assuredness, in your social poise, and possibly in future personal achievements. They will, in part, determine how other people respond to you, are attracted to you, and look up to you!

SOCIAL SUPPORTS

How a spouse/significant other, parents, friends, family members, teachers, and others care for us, listen to us, and treat us as an individual who matters can have a major impact on your self-worth and psychological adjustment. First and foremost, therefore, it is important to get your support network together (see chapter 1). Follow through on using that network. In doing so, you will get the support you need from people who know what you need because they've been there. You will also be able to give support to others who are in need. This gift alone will empower you and enhance your self-worth.

The support of your spouse/significant other and family is especially invaluable (see Chapter 10). Their support can be crucial to your well-being and can directly affect how you cope with scoliosis over time. Recognize that scoliosis may change roles within a family as regular household tasks become differently distributed among family members. Family members themselves need to accept this as a reality; they need to offer you the very support they might expect if they experienced a chronic health condition.

COPING WITH DAILY HASSLES

Decreasing daily hassles and negative life experiences can decrease adjustment problems and even your experience of symptoms. Here are suggestions for coping with a variety of scoliosis-related hassles such as brace-wear, surgery, household tasks, and the like.

BRACE-WEAR

Refer to chapter 2 as well as the following recommendations:

- Wear loose clothing for comfort and for deaccentuating rib humps.
- Wear a t-shirt under your brace so that the brace is not next to your skin. Bras can be uncomfortable under braces.
- Use moleskin strips over sore areas. These can be purchased at your pharmacy.
- High heels are uncomfortable. They are great for fashion, but not for your back.
- Don't carry things whenever possible. Try fanny packs or backpacks. Avoid things that hang from your shoulders.
- Braces can make holes in clothing. Cover screws and edges with tape or Band-Aids.

- Have two sets of school books: one set for school, and one for home.
- Consider adjustable and/or tilting desks.
- Sit on comfortable chairs. Softer is not necessarily better.
- Try prism glasses for TV viewing when lying down. Check with your optometrist about these.

General Coping

- Do regular physical exercise as prescribed by a physiatrist or physical therapist.
- Consider acupuncture, TENS or neuromuscular stimulators, and trigger point work. Ask your doctor about these approaches.
- Adjust computer angles properly. Use wrist supports. If you can, work from home using computer links.
- Treat yourself to a massage.
- Arrange furniture in the house with a logical flow. Buy furniture with the right height for your needs.
- Use an egg-crate mattress on your bed.
- Consider seat and back supports for a car or plane trip. Use medications appropriately, and take breaks when you can.
- Pay attention to your body when lifting.
- Install handles in your bath/shower for support.
- Consider a back support for dining out, at plays, movies, and amusement parks.
- Use a cart when shopping.
- Pace yourself. Don't overdo it. If you do, you'll know it.
- If you're buying a car, purchase one with good, firm seats and as many adjustments as you can afford—steering wheel angles, seat adjustments, power windows, lumbar supports, etc. Be sure you test drive a car before purchase.

Pre- and Post-Surgery

- Anticipate as much as you can *before* going to the hospital.
- Avoid bending, twisting, and carrying.
- Buy a long-handle reacher to grasp floor items—socks, shoes, any-

thing—to avoid bending.

- Use small containers vs. large ones for food storage, because they weigh less.
- Have a stool in your kitchen to lean your foot on. *Don't* use it for standing.
- Use an elevated toilet seat. Place toilet paper within your range of motion.
- Get a good chair for your back. Try it before you buy. The amount you spend may not correlate with the chair's comfort for *you*.
- Arrange kitchen shelves to avoid reaching, stretching, and lifting.
- Sit when you are dressing.
- Anchor your rugs to avoid slipping.
- Wear shoes that don't slip, especially in the rain.
- Buy an answering machine if you don't already have one. Screen your calls, then return calls when you feel up to it. Get a long extension cord to your phone, or use a cordless system.

CLOTHING ADJUSTMENTS

Clothing that fits properly can become a challenge for anyone with a physical deformity. For the person with scoliosis, it may mean trips to the tailor for an extra dart on a bodice to accommodate a thoracic hump. Or it may simply mean an adjustment to a hem to counteract a hip asymmetry. Whatever the need is, it is important to take care of it so you feel that you look good. When you look good, you feel good!

Two years ago, my mother and I were shopping for a special dress while on vacation. The dress I fell in love with buckled in the back where my right thoracic curve is. My mother could see the shock on my face. This is the first time my scoliosis became obvious to me—reality bites! My mother, quite nonchalantly, suggested that we have it altered to fit. We did, and all was well. However, from that point on ill-fitting clothes have become a fact of life for me. For my sixteenth birthday, my parents gave me a ballet tutu that was custom-designed by a well-known theatrical designer for my upcoming role as the Sugar Plum Fairy in the *Nutcracker*. I was to finally own my own scoli-tutu (as we called it). And, finally, I was able to wear a costume that fit me well. There's a solution to every problem.

CHAPTER 10

Every Patient Needs Support

Scoliosis is a chronic condition. That is, it continues to exist over weeks, months, and years. As such, it can be an ongoing stressor not only for the teenage patient, but also for his or her family—parents and siblings—who need to support the treatment plan over time.

PARENT REACTIONS

The initial diagnosis of scoliosis can have a significant emotional impact on parents. Although many parents take a rational and levelheaded public approach to the diagnosis, they may have many private feelings over time. Many parents experience disappointment, confusion, and anxiety. Others may feel anger, resentment, depression, and guilt. Some may feel little at first. This is usually due to the psychological mechanism of denial. Denial is an almost universal response to significant stressors. It is characterized by such thoughts as, "No, this can't be true" or "This isn't real" or "This information must be wrong—not my daughter/son." Denial may buffer intense feelings while giving parents a period of time to adjust to the information and may also be a first step on the path of acceptance and adjustment to any significant lifestyle changes that may need to follow.

Family Response Styles

Over time, families respond to the daily management of scoliosis in different ways, or styles. Some of these might include:

Balanced Style. In this style, parents take a healthy approach to the stresses of scoliosis. They are supportive, informed, and levelheaded. They are optimistic about treatment outcomes and encourage follow-through on prescribed regimens. Communication, consistency, and genuine caring characterize this style; it acknowledges scoliosis, but does not make it the focal point of the child's life.

Overanxious/Overprotective Style. In this style, parents and caregivers are overly influenced by their own anxieties, worries, and guilt. Their own concerns lead them to perceive their child as sick or delicate. They may hover over their child in a protective stance that can smother and restrict their child's personal and social development.

Overindulgent Style. In this approach, parents do not set adequate limits on their child, or are inconsistent with treatment follow-through. Perceiving their child as "needy," they give in to most of their child's wishes or shower him/her with presents, gifts, allowances, etc.

Overcontrolling/Rigid Style. In this style, parents follow treatment plans in an inflexible, dominating style. They attempt to control all areas of their child's life, even those having nothing to do with scoliosis. This diminishes their child's experience with self-direction and with learning the links between behaviors and their consequences.

Detached Style. In this approach, overwhelmed parents withdraw from their child's care and drop out of the caregiver role. They may reject their child and his/her situation, or become disinterested in and neglectful of their child's condition. Parental resentment, depression, and anger can contribute to this approach.

FAMILY FACTORS THAT CAN INFLUENCE RESPONSE STYLES

A number of factors contribute to the overall approach a family assumes to the management of scoliosis. They are as follows:

Communication. How well do we discuss and talk about family issues? Are we attuned to each other's needs?

Cohesiveness. How *supportive* and *together* are we when handling family stressors? Do we allow for independence in our approaches to problem solving?

Adaptability. How *flexible* and *resourceful* are we when facing problems? Do we know how to have fun, use our individual senses of humor, and focus on the positive?

Parent Interpersonal Factors. How loving and supportive are the mother and father towards each other? Are there marital conflicts? How do we cope with stress and pressures?

Surrounding Issues. Are there outside factors (*e.g.*, financial, job, schedules) generating stress for the family? Do we need to socialize with friends, and do we have an effective social support network?

Information. Do we have the information we need about scoliosis and its treatment? Should we explore other sources to find out how other people cope?

HOW TO ACHIEVE A BALANCED COPING STYLE IN THE FAMILY

Research indicates that the family of an individual with a diagnosed chronic condition may significantly influence the course of that condition, especially in terms of the distress, hopefulness, discomfort management, and disability status. As such, a balanced style of family coping can be quite important. Here are some suggestions on how to achieve it.

◆ Practice communication styles and ways of talking with each other that encourage hopefulness, support, and concern.

◆ Make sure that your viewpoint is reality-based and accurate. Try to avoid approaches to problems that catastrophize outcomes or are overly hysterical and emotional in their presentations.

◆ Allow for individuality and creativity in problem-solving. The old ways may not be the only ways to approach this new situation (scoliosis) for your family.

◆ Be consistent in the application of household "rules and regulations." An inconsistent and chaotic follow-through will not communicate limits and boundaries. Taking the time to set limits and to follow through on them means that you care.

◆ Use humor. Avoid sarcasm and personal insult, even if these approaches may get a laugh. Encourage a focus on attributes, not on perceived deficits.

◆ As a parent, be open to talking about the stresses that come from adhering to treatment plans such as bracing or the need for surgery. Be open to hearing about strong feelings such as anxiety, depression, and helplessness. Solve each issue one at a time.

◆ Set expectations that are realistic and can be achieved.

◆ Continue to view scoliosis as a part of the person and not as the whole person. There is more to life than scoliosis. Reframe issues to focus on capabilities rather than on limitations.

◆ Make sure your family has time for fun! Frequent fun activities can help to balance the stresses that result from chronic medical conditions. Practice personal stress management strategies.

◆ Develop and use a support network. Find out what others do or have done to cope. Accurate information will go a long way in easing anxiety.

◆ Don't let marital discord interfere with your child's scoliosis management. Be on the same wavelength as your spouse. If this is difficult, seek professional advice or counsel.

WHEN THE PATIENT IS YOUR WIFE, HUSBAND, OR SIGNIFICANT OTHER

The diagnosis of scoliosis in one's spouse and the real possibility of scoliosis surgery for that person can result in apprehension, anxiety, and emotional distress for the husband or significant other. The sources of distress can come from thoughts and fears about the following:

• Concerns about curve progression and its consequences.
• Concerns about the complexity of spinal fusion surgery and possible problematic outcomes.
• Seeing post-operative pain and discomfort in a loved one.
• Cosmetic or body appearance issues.
• Concerns about role-change issues after surgery (*e.g.*, from "breadwinner" to "family caretaker").
• Child care issues.
• Changes in family income resulting from a spouse's inability to work.
• Changes in sexual activity after surgery.

Scoliosis and its surgical management can affect many interacting areas in a relationship, all at the same time. These issues can be stressful and can result in many conflicting feelings for the spouse/partner of the patient. Love, compassion, fear, frustration, resentment, and anger may all coexist. Many spouse/partners may not know how to express these feelings. Some feel guilty about having these feelings, given the magnitude of their loved one's surgical experience.

SUGGESTIONS FOR SPOUSE/PARTNERS

The issues just discussed require a range of coping skills. Here are some suggestions a spouse or significant other may find helpful, whether or not surgery is required.

◆ Accept the fact that scoliosis and/or its surgical management is not just your partner's problem. As previously indicated, you may have several areas in your life disrupted as well. Recognizing this will give you the openness and opportunity to prepare for what lies ahead.

◆ Inform yourself. Find out all you can about scoliosis and its management. Find out about the surgery, both in its pre- and post-operative phases. Ask the surgeon any and all questions you may have. Read current books and other publications on scoliosis. The more facts you have, the better prepared you will be. The fewer surprises, the better.

◆ Talk to other spouses about their experiences. You can do this by joining local scoliosis support chapters. You and your partner should *both* join. This way, you can both ask questions of people who have "been there." Many support chapters have regular presentations by surgeons and other allied health professionals, which will help you be on top of the latest information. You also won't feel so alone or overwhelmed.

◆ Accurately evaluate the information you have. Avoid ways of thinking that lead you to see only negative outcomes, or permit you to see only the worst. Avoid catastrophizing. By contrast, saying things like, "Everything's going to be all right" and "Let the pros handle everything" without your input and personal planning may put you and your partner in an even more vulnerable position if problems arise, simply because you are not prepared for them. Try to keep a balanced outlook on surgery and its outcome.

◆ Recognize that scoliosis surgery may cause temporary changes in sexual relations. Some sexual activities may need modification. You may want to try different positions or to change roles from more to less active, or vice versa. Creative ways of sexual expression may need to be explored during the recuperation process. Communication at this time is very important.

◆ Talk about how you feel. Many men find this extremely difficult to do. They often have not grown up accepting their emotions, and do not have much experience discussing them. This is simply a product of the society in which we live. Unfortunately, bottling up feelings and keeping them unexpressed is not healthy during this stressful time.

Try to talk to your partner first of all about how *he or she* feels. Be prepared to hear words like "scared," "worried," and "anxious." Acknowledge these feelings and accept them. Don't dismiss them. Then, tell her how *you* feel. You'll probably find you are using many of the same words. Conversations like this can bring you closer to each other during this mutually stressful time. You may actually be each other's best support system.

If you find you don't want to talk to other people face-to-face, a computer may be the way to go for you. There is plenty of information on-line on a variety of web pages, medical support bulletin boards, Usenet newsgroups, etc. You can find less intimate ways of "talking" to people via e-mail and chat rooms. This is becoming a very viable option for many men. However, it is not a substitute for meaningful conversations with your partner.

◆ Plan ahead. Get your support systems in place before you need them. Can anyone help you when your partner comes home from the hospital? What about child care? Can family or friends help with cooking or other routine tasks for awhile? This is reasonable preplanning that will reduce your stress during a difficult time.

◆ Try to continue with effective stress management strategies you already use. If you work out, try to continue to do so. Pressures may change your routines, so modify your schedule but try not to give your routines up completely. Avoid increases in alcohol use. Although alcohol may provide some temporary relief, it does not allow you to feel your best physically and can negatively affect how you handle emotional strains and pressures in the long run.

Many couples say that "weathering the storm" of scoliosis and of major surgery has brought them closer together. For others, these pressures put undue stress on their relationship. This might be true for a couple in a new relationship or those in marriages with pre-existing discord. If this is true for you, seek professional advice and support. The skills you learn can help greatly to offset the pressures you will be facing.

WHEN THE PATIENT IS A PARENT

Sometimes scoliosis can cause chronic pain and fatigue, which can also have an impact on your children. However, from a child's point of view, scoliosis in a parent is probably most evident when that parent, usually Mom, requires surgery. Major surgery for a parent needing a significant hospital stay and with an extended recuperation period at home will result in a major disruption in daily living. The focus of parental attention will shift, household routines will change, and many daily events will likely become uncertainties for an indefinite period of time.

How these changes are experienced can depend on the age of your child. Older children and teens with life experiences and independence may be less affected than the younger child who is quite dependent. As such, although the separation resulting from the hospital stay is difficult for all family members, younger children have fewer life experiences and a reduced life context through which to interpret an event such as surgery. Younger children are quite concrete in their understanding of life events (out of sight means literally "gone" and "out of mind"—Piaget's idea of irreversibility) and so these children may need special attention in order to deal with anxiety resulting from Mom's hospital stay.

Here are some suggestions for talking to your child about Mom or Dad's hospitalization and surgery:

♦ Try to understand this experience from your child's point of view. How old is he or she? Can he/she understand what surgery is? Explain it, if necessary, in terms that your child can understand. (Example: "Mom's back really hurts. A very good doctor is going to fix it. She will be in the hospital for a little while, and she will be home as soon as she feels better".) The older child may ask more detailed questions. Tailor your answers to their age and level of sophistication.

♦ Tell your child what to expect. Most fears at this time come from not knowing what to expect. Discuss what the surgery involves in terms of what your child needs to know. Older teens can generally tolerate details. Younger children need to know that Mom or Dad will be "fixed" and that everything will be okay.

◆ Answer questions honestly. Be prepared for direct and concrete questions from younger children. (Example: "Can Mom take care of us after the operation?" or "Why won't all her blood leak out?") Let your teen know that you will need his or her help. Involve him/her in the preparations for post-surgery.

◆ Tell children that someone they trust will always be available. Have a support network in place. This will significantly reduce your child's anxiety. It is better if close relatives and friends can be enlisted for this task. The more familiar, trusted, and consistent your helpers are, the better.

◆ Recognize and understand your children's feelings and emotions. Concerns regarding personal safety, post-surgical discomfort, and a secure tomorrow may be unspoken issues. Address them before they arise.

◆ Be clear that Mom or Dad will return from the hospital as soon as the doctor decides that she or he is okay. This is especially important for younger children to understand.

◆ Be consistent in your availability to offer loving support despite your many demands and pressures at this time.

◆ Be aware that younger children may need extra attention with a parent's absence. Some backward behavioral steps might be seen during this period of emotional distress (*e.g.*, bedwetting, thumb sucking, jealousy among siblings, etc.). This is okay. The passage of time will help to heal and normalize this difficult experience. A sense of accomplishment and personal pride may result from the family's progress through this trying period together.

CHAPTER 11

Building Self-Esteem

What home environments foster self-esteem in teenagers? Research suggests the importance of three conditions. First, that parents communicate their *acceptance* of teens—that teens know they belong in the family and are prized and valued members. Second, that parents communicate *well-defined limits* and *expectations for performance*. As such, teenagers recognize the expectations for mature behavior and their parents' confidence in their abilities. (Of course, expectations should be reasonable and appropriate for the child's age.) Third, that parents *respect* the teenager's *individuality*, allowing him/her the latitude to be different and unique within generally established boundaries. Teenagers' observations of their own parents' self-esteem and of their approaches to handling challenges, difficulties, and disappointments can also influence the teen's sense of confidence and a sense of efficacy in meeting life's challenges. As such, parents can be teachers and models for attitudes in their children that are optimistic, coping-oriented, self-supportive, and nonself-critical.

What are the signs and symptoms that a teenager may be experiencing self-esteem problems? Many teenagers accept the diagnosis of scoliosis and possible bracing requirements. Others may have difficulty. Clues to difficulties may come from expressed (or private) apprehensions, worry and anxiety, self-critical statements, concerns about the future, avoidance of social situations and friends, depression, frustration, anger, and thoughts about body image. Falling school grades, various physical complaints, changes in eating or sleeping habits, and irritability and moodiness may accompany self-esteem-based problems. Parents need to be aware of average or "baseline" behaviors and statements from their children in order to detect changes that might occur.

CONSIDERATIONS FOR IMPROVING SELF-ESTEEM

People with low self-esteem are often pathological self-critics. They blame themselves for everything that goes wrong, compare themselves to others (and find themselves wanting), or set impossible standards of perfection for themselves and then beat themselves up for the inevitable smallest mistake. Their self-criticism regularly undermines their self-worth. What's more, this self-criticism often seems reasonable and justified to the person! In the frequency of occurrence, these criticisms form the fabric of an "I am not okay" viewpoint of themselves in daily interactions. What can parents do? Fortunately, there are several approaches:

◆ Make sure your teenager *accurately* assesses his/her strengths and shortcomings. People with low self-esteem do not see themselves clearly. They magnify their own weaknesses and minimize their assets. Furthermore, they usually describe their weaknesses in the most pejorative ways. "Stupid," "fat," and "ugly" are routine self-descriptors for these individuals. Parents can help their teenagers to remember their strengths and to celebrate them actively! They can help their teenagers to challenge negative self-talk with appropriate questions such as, "What is the evidence for that?" or "Are you looking at both or all sides of the issue?" Parents can help teenagers counter negative inner dialogue by developing a list of accurate, positive, self-supportive statements. These may include affirmations about loveability, capability, and self-acceptance, as well as what your teen is learning from daily living. "I am learning to do things I never thought I was capable of doing" or "I may have scoliosis, but that doesn't mean I am any less of a person," are just two of many possibilities. Affirmations must be used regularly to disrupt and to replace chains of negative thoughts. Other examples of affirmations might include:

- I am a valuable and important person.
- I am worthy of the respect of others.
- I am optimistic about life. I have a positive outlook on the future.
- I feel warm and loving toward myself. I am a unique and precious person.
- By wearing the brace/having surgery, I am in charge of my scoliosis treatment.
- I am an active contributor to my health and well-being.

By the same token, it is important for parents to see their child as he/she *really* is. Accurately seeing your children helps build self-esteem several ways:

- You are able to recognize their unique abilities and talents—to reinforce them, nurture them, and to help them recognize what is special about themselves.
- You are able to understand their behavior in the context of *who they are* (not who they remind you of, or how they ought to be, or hope they should be).
- It helps you to focus on behaviors that are important to change, such as harmful, isolative, or disruptive behaviors. This helps to avoid needless criticism of personal tastes, styles, and preference.
- Teenagers who feel they are really seen and understood by their parents can afford to be themselves. They don't have to hide parts of themselves because they fear rejection. If you can accept all of your child, both the good and the bad, your child can accept all of himself/herself. This is the foundation of good self-esteem.

◆ Create an atmosphere of comfort and acceptance at home. Some suggestions here might be: work together, express affection, relax and enjoy one another, have family and friends visit often, keep plants or flowers in the house, share stories together, give compliments, and say, "I love you" more often. Share ideas with your child on what a happy home is like, and act on some of these ideas more often. This will help your child understand that scoliosis is a *part* of his/her life; it does not have to be the focus of his/her life.

◆ Beware of cognitive distortions in your teen's communications. Cognitive distortions are actually bad habits—habits of thought—that are consistently used to interpret reality in an inaccurate and unreal way. They are generally judgmental. They automatically apply labels to the individual, other people, and events with little regard for balance, truthfulness, accuracy, or rationality. Here are some distortions that undermine self-esteem:

- *Overgeneralization*—With this distortion, we come to a general conclusion based on a single incident or piece of evidence. Key distortion words are: never, always, all, every, none, nobody, everybody. For example, "*Nobody* will accept me," "*Everybody* will think I'm awkward (or stupid, or ugly, etc.)," or "I'll *never* be able to do this." To counter these statements, ask, "What are the odds of this reality being true?" and "Has this been true in the past?" Help your child to compare his/her statements with positive experiences and accomplishments in his/her past.

- *Global labeling*—This is the application of stereotyped labels to whole classes of people, things, behaviors, and experiences. Examples are: "I am a failure," "I look totally ugly." To counter, get rid of words like failure, stupid, clumsy, ugly, hopeless. Replace the label with a balanced, accurate definition.

- *Filtering*—Here, negative details are magnified, while all positive aspects of a situation are filtered out. It's as dangerous to self-esteem as piloting an airplane with your eyes closed! Whenever you notice it, ask, "Am I looking at the whole picture?" and "Are there any positive aspects of this situation that I am ignoring?" Look for the opposite of what you filter for. For example, "Maybe I can't do everything I used to do before wearing the brace, but I'm learning to overcome a lot of obstacles," or "Maybe I don't look or feel my best now, but if I stick with the treatment, maybe I can avoid surgery, and look better after treatment."

- *Self-blame*—This is a distorted thinking style that has a person blaming himself/herself for everything, whether or not he/she was actually at fault. The blame is for everything—like being sick, thinking you are responsible for your parents' divorce, having scoliosis, or whatever. To counter, *rigorously* weed out judgmental statements and replace them with balanced ones.

- *"Should" statements*—"Shoulds" are ironclad rules about how we and others must act. They are at the core of value systems for many of us. They often develop in response to basic personal needs, or the need to feel belonging and approval from peers, or are acquired from parents, teachers, or other authority persons. "Shoulds" often tyrannize the lives of those with low self-esteem: "I should be perfect," "I should never have gotten scoliosis," "I should never be sick," "I should never be afraid," "I should be loved by everyone." All of these (and many more) can set standards that are inflexible, life-restricting, and unrealistic. To counter, notice when words like should or must are being used. Evaluate the standards as healthy, flexible, realistic, and life-enhancing. If not, cut them out of the internal or external dialogue. Replace them with healthier beliefs, values, and personal rules. Values that include a tolerance of oneself and a sense of self-compassion (not self-pity) are particularly helpful for building positive self-esteem.

◆ Examine communication styles in your home. Communication at home is essential for your teenager's self-esteem. When you stop and listen to your child, you communicate your interest and caring. You are saying, "You are important. What you say matters to me. *You* matter to me." Yet, the pressures of daily living compete for our attention. How can we listen better?

- Make sure you have *the time* to really listen. Try to set aside time just for talking to your teen. Even if it's for ten minutes, give your child your full attention. Be there, fully present. Shut off the distractions. If your teen is telling you something personal, find a private place to talk.

- Be an active listener. Ask questions, clarify situations, respond, and look at your child. Give cues that you are interested. Remember names of friends and teachers. Ask for updates on the previous day's concerns. Your child will feel important if you remember what's important to him/her.

- Invite your child to talk. Even if your teen doesn't demand your attention, he/she may still need it. Make a special time together devoted to him/her alone. Ask some open-ended question, then follow your child's need. Avoid criticism about school grades, the messy room, or matters of style and preference.

◆ What do you listen for?
   • Listen for the point of the story. Ask yourself, "What is he/she trying to tell me?" or "What is the reason this is important to him/her?" Is this about a success? Is he/she embarrassed, or angry, or confused? Give feedback to the *point of the story*, and not to the flood of details that might accompany it.
   • Don't feel you have to fix everything. Sometimes you just have to listen. You don't have to make suggestions, give advice, or solve the problem. Often, giving "the solution" actually cuts the other person off. Remember, sometimes your teen needs to share an experience or simply ventilate feelings. Also, it's important to help your child come up with his/her own solutions to various problems. This will do more for his/her self-esteem than if you impose "the fix." Remember, too, that many problems don't have obvious solutions, or at least none that are evident until feelings are expressed and aired.
   • Listen and respond to feelings. Try not only to listen to the words, but to the feelings underneath the words. What does this posture or tone of voice mean? Is he/she excited or happy, or disappointed and dejected? Look for the cues that communicate the feelings. They are a vital part of most communications. Losing touch with feelings, denying their existence, repressing them, or ridiculing them can only diminish self-esteem. Be a good role model in how you deal with your own strong feelings. Share some of your coping skills with your teenager. Also, don't forget to praise your child for a job well done, for a difficulty that's over, or a challenge that has been met. Your approval shapes behavior. When you praise your teen, he/she gets the message that he/she is okay, and that what he/she does is acceptable and appreciated.

A consistent application of these concepts and strategies can go a long way toward enhancing a teenager's self-esteem. Acceptance of diagnosis, active participation in treatment, his/her level of coping, and ability to feel good about himself/herself depend on it!

Sometimes, the "not okay" feelings can be extremely difficult to overcome. If you have tried the approach we recommend, and the issues still remain, don't give up hope! Many people require the help of a trained psychotherapist to help change long-standing negative feelings. The support of another person who is caring and who has the knowledge to help can be invaluable in facilitating movement through the change process. Don't be afraid to ask for that help.

SCOLIOSIS AND SEX

Scoliosis, in and of itself, usually has a minimal effect on the physiology and mechanics of sex. However, issues associated with the management of scoliosis over time, such as self-image and body image, the trauma of one or more major surgeries, or coping with chronic pain may have a significant impact on a person's thoughts and feelings about intimacy and sexuality. Let's take a look at these issues from a few different points in the lifespan, with an eye toward developing healthy perspectives on sex and sexuality.

TEENAGERS

Although having sex is not an issue for all teenagers, it is a concern for many. Some estimates indicate that sixty percent of adolescents between the ages of fifteen and nineteen are sexually active, and seventy-nine percent of undergraduate college students have engaged in sexual intercourse. As such, thoughts and feelings about sex and sexuality are prominent in the lives of teenagers.

If you are a teenager, you probably have many thoughts about dating and sex. You are probably quite concerned with your own physical appearance and how your peers notice and respond to you. You are probably aware of how other teenagers deal with issues of dating and sex, and you may be wondering how you fit in. What you see on television, in the movies, or on the Internet regarding sexuality may be a bit confusing. Whether you do or don't have a boyfriend/girlfriend, you may feel pressured to do things before you are ready to do them. On top of all this, you may have recently been diagnosed as having scoliosis. You may need to wear a brace. It is normal to have concerns about how scoliosis and bracing will affect your physical appearance. Many wonder if their peers will be turned off by physical appearance with or without brace wear. Some girls wonder if the brace will restrict their breast development. Some may wonder, "How can I feel sexy or even think about having sex when I have scoliosis and I'm wearing this thing?" Here are some suggestions:

◆ It is *very* important for you to have someone you can talk to about thoughts, concerns, and fears regarding physical appearance and sexuality. Just having someone listen to you, without judging, validates you and helps you to feel better about yourself. You also need to have facts. Don't be afraid or embarrassed to ask your doctor any and all questions you may have. If necessary, ask your parents if you can have a few minutes privately with your doctor during your scheduled appointment. Correct and accurate information is what you need. Unanswered questions or those that you may feel too awkward to ask can loom larger than life in your thoughts. For some people, unanswered questions can become real worries, which restrict daily living. Don't let this happen to you.

◆ Try talking to your parents about your concerns. If you do not feel you are able to talk with either or both of them, by all means, talk to a good friend. Feedback can be quite useful. Consider talking to a school psychologist or guidance counselor. See if there is a scoliosis support group in your area that has teenage members. Often, the teenagers meet in a small group by themselves, which is a great opportunity to share concerns and exchange ideas with others who know *exactly* what you're talking about.

◆ Don't isolate yourself. Some teenagers who are afraid of rejection by others solve the problem by withdrawing and remaining alone. This is rarely a good solution in the long run and can make the immediate situation more lonely and painful. Stay connected with friends and remain as active as you can. The bigger your support network, the better.

◆ Avoid words like "never," "no," and "nobody" in your thinking. Thoughts such as "*No* guy/girl will like me," or "I'll *never* be attractive with this condition," or "*Nobody* will find me sexy" distort your reality and only make you feel worse about your situation and yourself. How you think and feel about yourself is every bit as (and *more*) important than how others evaluate you.

Having a negative view of your future only hurts your self-esteem in the present. This, in turn, will lessen the poise and self-confidence you need to project to others—the very things that make you attractive! So don't sabotage yourself with negative future thinking. Don't anticipate the worst. Take things one step at a time—in reality and in the present.

For Parents

Most parents do not have an easy time thinking about or discussing their child's/teenager's dating and sexuality concerns. Yet, as statistics tell us, sex is a very real part of our teenager's world. Those who have scoliosis and who need to wear a brace are particularly vulnerable to feelings of "standing out and being different," to self-image and body-image concerns, and to sexual inadequacy worries. As such, even though your daughter/son may appear to be unconcerned and may not wish to discuss this topic, the chances are that this is an upfront, underlying concern. Here are some thoughts and suggestions:

◆ Make yourself available to talk with your teenager about sexual issues. Some studies suggest that less than twenty percent of parents actually do this despite the fact that teenagers would like to talk to their parents about sexual concerns. You should prepare yourself with accurate information about sexual matters and by thinking through your own values in these matters beforehand. Your teenager may like to know how *you* arrived at your personal values on sexual behavior.

◆ If your teenager isn't asking questions or expressing concerns about sexual issues and scoliosis and/or brace wear, be proactive and ask some questions. Don't be misled into believing that "She's only twelve and isn't concerned about that," or "My kid doesn't worry about that stuff." He/she may simply be too embarrassed or afraid that you will misjudge her/him. Practice good, honest, open communication if these sexual matters don't surface in daily interaction.

◆ Listen carefully to what your teenager says. Although most teenagers with scoliosis follow a normal path of healthy adjustment, some who are wearing a brace may feel seriously unattractive, that they look like outer space creatures, that surgery will disfigure them, and that no one will want to have sex with them. They may feel depressed and even desperate. If you hear words like, "Life is meaningless" or "It's just no use," your child may be having a much harder time than you first thought. Keep communication open. Get professional advice if your teenager remains depressed about these important issues over a period of time. Themes of sadness, helplessness, and hopelessness need to be taken seriously.

Adults Facing Surgery

If you are an adult facing surgery, you may have many questions and concerns about the effects of spinal fusion surgery on sexual activity. Many of these fears may harken back to your own teenage feelings about rejection, unacceptability, inadequacy, and intimacy. You may be thinking, "Will sex be painful after the operation?" or "Will my husband look at me in the same way?" or "Will I be able to use the same positions? Will they be comfortable?" or "Will I be able to feel sexy? Wear sexy clothes? Look pretty and attractive?" or "Will I be able to have a normal pregnancy if I decide to have a child?" or "Will I be able to lift and carry an infant and toddler, as well as baby accessories?" We suggest the following:

◆ Talk to your doctor about your sexual concerns. She or he will probably tell you that you can resume sexual activity when you feel ready after surgery, but that some positions may need to be modified for awhile during your recuperation. Ask your doctor any and all questions you may have about pregnancy and scoliosis. Ask your surgeon to refer you to other patients your age who have had the surgery and had a child afterwards. This way, you will have accurate information to counter your fears and concerns.

◆ Talk to your spouse/significant other about your sexual concerns. If you have spoken to your doctor, or other women your age who have had the surgery, you probably have the information we just discussed. Keep open and honest communication with your spouse. If, after surgery, some sexual positions are uncomfortable, talk about this with your spouse. Be creative in your approach to

sexual expression and behavior. You may discover some pleasant
activities you hadn't thought of before!

◆ As we've said elsewhere, join local support groups. This will put
you in direct contact with others who are coping with or who
have already been through a similar situation. You will get the
information and reassurance you need at this time.

CHRONIC PAIN AND SEXUAL ACTIVITY

If you are experiencing chronic discomfort and pain, you are probably
well aware of how such pain can make you feel less attractive and less
confident in areas related to sex and sexuality. You may have feelings of
resentment, frustration, anger, or depression about your scoliosis and
how it has affected your sexual activity and interest. You may also be
concerned about the effects of your feelings on your spouse and on your
sexual relationship with him/her.

In chapter 9, we discussed a biopsychosocial strategy for coping with
chronic pain in general. These are some specific suggestions for coping
with chronic pain and discomfort in sexual activity:

◆ Accept and acknowledge the negative feelings you may have about
your pain and sexual activity. Acceptance is a first step toward
working through and getting beyond these feelings.

◆ Communicate with your spouse/significant other about your feelings and discomfort. Find the time to talk frankly, honestly, and
gently about the sexual needs and ideas you both may have. This
may be an important step toward exploring new and satisfying sexual activities. Develop a signal system that lets your spouse/partner
know when you are in pain or when a certain activity is too
uncomfortable to continue.

◆ Consider planning for sex at a time of day when you know you
feel your best. Although spontaneous sex can be great, if it occurs
when you are in pain or fatigued, it may be less satisfying for you
and your partner. Planning for sex can also allow you to pace your
activity throughout a given day.

◆ Try taking a warm shower or bath before sex. Not only is this important for personal grooming, it might help you to feel less achy or stiff during sex. A gentle massage before sex can also be helpful in increasing flexibility. It may enhance your interest in sexual activity as well.

◆ If you take pain medication, time your dosage (if you can) for maximum effectiveness during sex. Discuss the possible use of antidepressants with your doctor. Antidepressants (as discussed in chapter 9) can raise your pain threshold and your interest in sexual activity. However, you should be aware that some antidepressants, while raising your pain threshold, also inhibit your ability to have an orgasm. Discuss possible side effects with your doctor.

◆ Consider different positions for sexual intercourse. Different positions may put less stress on your back and may allow for more or less movement on your part, thereby increasing satisfaction and decreasing effort. Sometimes chronic pain can decrease vaginal lubrication. Some medications can also have this effect. Use a vaginal lubricant (not petroleum jelly) to facilitate enjoyment in different lovemaking positions.

◆ If sexual intercourse is not okay at certain times, consider manual sex as a way of lovemaking. Gently carressing each other's bodies and touching sensitive body areas can be a satisfying approach to lovemaking. Oral sex can be an exciting substitute for or complement to more traditional ways of sexual expression.

◆ Masturbation or self-stimulation can be a healthy and satisfying way of sexual expression. Taking the time to explore one's body and sensitive body areas can result in greater sexual responsiveness. It can also help a person with chronic discomfort know what does or does not feel good in sexual activity.

CHAPTER 12

Searching for the Genetic Cause

Happiness, as my mother pointed out, might be
good health and a short memory, but what do we
do with the genetic memory which is inescapable?
—Isabella Rossellini, *Some of Me*

I was profoundly affected by this question raised by Ingrid Bergman at the time of her daughter Isabella's scoliosis surgery. Today, more than thirty years later, the subject of "genetic memory" remains a mystery in the etiology of idiopathic scoliosis. At the time of my own diagnosis, the initial shock and dismay experienced by my family and me was quickly followed by such questions as "where did this come from?" "from whom did I get it?" and "am I the only one in the whole family who has it?" For the next three years I was to hear these very questions expressed by the hundreds of people I had the privilege of meeting through my toll-free phone number and my travels. In some cases a family member may be identifiable: a grandmother with a hunched over posture no one ever questioned, a cousin who walked with a limp because of a hip asymmetry, or an uncle who displayed an obvious raised shoulder. In other cases there can be no identifiable trace of scoliosis history. While scoliosis is often a secondary condition to other predisposing disorders and diseases (see sidebar), eighty-five percent (between two and three percent of the adolescent population) of all scoliosis is idiopathic and, therefore, naturally raises the question of genetics.

Although the specific cause has not yet been identified, it is widely accepted that genetics plays a large role. Thus family inheritance is

SCOLIOSIS SECONDARY TO AN UNDERLYING DISEASE

CEREBRAL PALSY

Significant structural deformities of the spine are often associated with cerebral palsy. Scoliosis is the most common of these spinal deformities. Treatment for the cerebral palsy patient is largely dependent upon the degree of curvature, patient's age, presence of symptoms and functional impairment.

POLIO

While polio is not as common today as it was decades ago, there still exist people who suffer from this affliction of yesteryear. The incidence of scoliosis in these patients varies depending upon the type and severity of musculature involved. Double major thoracic-lumbar curves are the most common. Again, as with the cerebral palsy patient, the treatment of scoliosis in the polio patient is largely dependent upon the severity of the curves, functional impairment, symptoms, and respiratory compromise.

MUSCULAR DYSTROPHY

The most common of all dystrophies is the Duchenne Muscular Dystrophy. The incidence of progressive scoliosis as a secondary condition in these patients is 90 to 95 percent. The natural history of scoliosis in muscular dystrophy patients is progression; this progression is most prevalent after the loss of walking ability in patients. Treatment with a brace seems to be ineffective in these patients; surgery is the mainstay of treatment for the Duchenne Muscular Dystrophy patient.

MARFAN'S SYNDROME

A person with Marfan's Syndrome will generally present a tall, slender build with disproportionately long arms, legs, fingers, and toes. Spinal deformity occurs in approximately 75 percent of these patients; the majority of spinal deformity cases are double ("S" shaped) curves.

The development of scoliosis in a Marfan's Syndrome patient usually occurs early in life (before the age of ten). The curves that these patients exhibit are similar to those of idiopathic scoliosis patients in that they are quick to progress during adolescence. Bracing treatment is often used as an effective way to stabilize the spine for patients who will eventually require surgery. Surgical treatment is indicated for progressive curves of forty-five to fifty degrees in the adolescent Marfan's Syndrome patient, or for painful, progressive curves of measurements greater than fifty degrees in the adult.

NEUROFIBRAMATOSIS

Scoliosis is the most common musculoskeletal complication associated with neurofibramatosis. The curves in these patients are typically short and sharp, usually involving six vertebrae or fewer. Typical idiopathic curves can also manifest themselves in neurofibramatosis patients; these curves can be treated as would any normal, idiopathic scoliosis.

observed, though the pattern of inheritance and susceptibility is not clear. Much research is being done around the world conducting population studies specifically focused on families with a high incidence of documented scoliosis.

In the spring of 1998, a worldwide group of researchers convened at the Philip Zorab International Scoliosis Conference in Oxford, England. The genetics group included researchers from the United States, Canada, Japan, and the United Kingdom, and announced the following conclusions:

- "the majority of families fit more into a complex trait or multi-factorial mode of inheritance"
- "it has reduced penetrance and variable expressivity"
- "the severity . . . within families can change and sometimes generations are skipped"[30]

Studies from the United States and Russia conclude that hereditary ideopathic scoliosis is an autosomal dominant trait, which means it can be inherited from either parent. These studies record an incomplete penetrance of the disorder—that is, two people with similar scoliosis genes do not necessarily show the same symptoms—and a sex bias toward females.

In addition to genetic studies, much research has focused on other possible causative agents for scoliosis, such as growth. Human growth involves a complex interaction with genetics, hormones, and environment. Hormonal studies have implicated an increased release of growth hormone in adolescent idiopathic scoliosis, though findings are not consistently reproduced. Analysis of connective tissue in adolescent idiopathic scoliosis patients and a control group showed some qualitative and quantitative variations. But other studies have shown that changes and differences in collagen types in adolescents compared to adults may be the result of the spinal deformity and not the cause of it.

Posture reflexes in adolescent scoliosis is another area which has been studied extensively. Scoliotics and non-scoliotics have been tested with techniques including labyrinthine stimulation and electroencephalograph (EEG). Scoliotics were observed to have increased postural sway compared to the controls.

The role of melatonin deficiency in experimental scoliosis in chickens has also been extensively researched in the etiology of idiopathic scoliosis. The conclusion was that melatonin deficiency interferes with the normal development of the proprioceptive system and spinal musculature, an etiologic factor in adolescent and idiopathic scoliosis. Clinical studies have confirmed decreased melatonin levels in patients with idiopathic scoliosis. However, other studies have also shown no difference in urinary melatonin levels in a clinical study of patients with idiopathic scoliosis and control subjects, indicating that melatonin deficiency may not be a causative agent in idiopathic scoliosis.

In summary, all of the study results imply that the cause of adolescent idiopathic scoliosis is multifactorial, involving a complex interplay of genetic, neuromuscular, and hormonal factors. For now, scoliosis cannot be prevented—it is all the more important, then, to make sure children are screened by trained observers so that treatment can begin while the spine still has time to grow.

The natural history, physiology and clinical outcomes for adult scoliosis differ greatly from adolescent scoliosis. Scoliosis may be present at the onset of adulthood from preexisting adolescent scoliosis, or may develop during adulthood in a previously straight spine. This can result from a metabolic bone disease such as osteothorosis or osteomalacia. The prevalence of this kind of condition is four percent for lumbar curves measuring more than ten degrees.

Though we may be frustrated in our concern for today's children, we can feel more encouraged as we educate ourselves and those around us regarding the latest research being done. Most of the studies cited conclude that a more accurate interpretation of the complex causes of scoliosis will only be possible as more patients with the disorder come forward. Also, international collaboration has already proven to be successful and is deemed necessary to expedite the sharing of information to find the cause of scoliosis.

Together we can defeat this disorder called scoliosis. As Stanley Sacks has written in the journal *Backtalk*, "[Doctors and scoliosis support groups are] joining researchers worldwide. If you or members of your family have scoliosis, you can help advance the important work of a gene identification. Let's look forward together to a day of better treatments and even prevention of this [disorder] affecting so many of our loved ones."[31]

Resource Directory

AMERICAN ACADEMY OF ORTHOPAEDIC SURGEONS
BACK PAIN HOTLINE (800) 824-BONES

A public service line available twenty-four hours a day. You may call to receive any of the free publications such as *Lift it Safe*, *Prevent Back Pain*, and *Keep Moving for Life*, which include tips for coping with back pain.

ARTHRITIS FOUNDATION
(800) 283-7800

Available twenty-four hours a day. A nonprofit organization that provides information on arthritis such as strategies for pain management, current treatment, exercises, and self-help methods. You can receive brochures, physician referrals, and other helpful information for adults and children.

NATIONAL INSURANCE CONSUMER HELPLINE
(800) 942-4242

Available 8:00 A.M. to 8:00 P.M. Eastern Time, Monday through Friday. Funded by the Insurance Information Institute, the American Council of Life Insurance, and the Health Insurance Association of America. This helpline will answer questions regarding different types of insurance. Brochures available.

NATIONAL MARFAN FOUNDATION
(800) 8-MARFAN

Available 8:00 A.M. to 3:30 P.M. Eastern Time, Monday through Friday. A nonprofit organization that "serves the needs of people with Marfan Syndrome and related connective tissue disorders." It provides free informational mailings and literature and online access via electronic mail and a web site on the Internet, www.marfan.org. There are chapters throughout the country which act as support groups. This organization holds an annual conference which is open to the public and health professionals.

NATIONAL NEUROFIBRAMATOSIS FOUNDATION
(800) 323-7938

Available 9:00 A.M. to 5:00 P.M. Eastern Time, Monday through Friday. A nonprofit organization that provides information, pamphlets, and referrals upon request. Its main mission is to facilitate research to treat and cure NF 1 and NF 2. Thirty-two chapters nationwide provide support and information and take part in fund-raising for research.

RELAX THE BACK STORE
(914) 472-BACK

"The Best Of Everything For Your Back." Call to inquire about pillows, chairs, and other mechanisms that will make living with back pain a lot easier.

SCOLIOSIS ASSOCIATION, INC.
(800) 800-0669

A nonprofit support organization designed to help patients and families cope with the physical, emotional and social problems related to having scoliosis. Its nationwide chapters provide information to educate the public about scoliosis, raise funds for scoliosis research, and provide peer support and physician referral. It publishes *Backtalk*, which features articles of interest from leading specialists on research and treatment of scoliosis, every two months. Website: www.scoliosis-assoc.org

SCOLIOSIS FOUNDATION
(617) 341-6333

A nonprofit organization that provides information to help children, adults, families and healthcare providers with the complexities of spinal deformities such as scoliosis. It promotes awareness and education in the scoliosis community, while fund-raising for ongoing research.

SCOLIOSIS RESEARCH SOCIETY
(847) 698-1627

An administrative organization for *doctors only*, this prestigious society is made up of surgeons who specialize in scoliosis. The SRS promotes research into the management and treatment of scoliosis. While the SRS is not a physician referral source, they will reveal which scoliosis surgeons in your state are members of their organization. Website: www.srs.org

SHRINERS' HOSPITALS
(800) 237-5055

Nineteen orthopedic Shriners' Hospitals across the country offer state-of-the-art medical care to children (ages eighteen and under) with problems of the bones, joints, or muscles. Admission is based on medical and financial need.

SPINA BIFIDA ASSOCIATION OF AMERICA
(800) 621-3141

Available 9:00 A.M. to 5:00 P.M. Eastern Time, Monday through Friday; answering machine after hours. Nationwide chapters provide information on educational programs, legislation, research, and public awareness. Several publications available.

SPONDYLITIS ASSOCIATION OF AMERICA
(800) 777-8189

Available 9:00 A.M. to 5:00 P.M. Pacific Time, Monday through Friday. After hours answering machine is available. A nonprofit organization that "helps people affected by ankylosing spondylitis and related diseases to lead productive lives, to familiarize health care professionals with early symptoms and appropriate treatments, and to fund research to discover the cause and find a cure." Website: www.spondylitis.org

VISITING NURSE ASSOCIATION OF AMERICA
(800) 426-2547

Available 7:00 A.M. TO 6:00 P.M. Central Time, Monday through Friday; answering machine after hours. This national toll-free referral line puts callers in touch with community-based nonprofit home healthcare organizations in their area. Services include general nursing, physical, occupational and speech therapy, and a host of other specialties.

Glossary

Adams forward bending test. A routine test to screen for scoliosis used by school nurses and doctors. The patient bends from the waist with arms stretched forward and hands clasped.

Adolescent scoliosis. A three-dimensional spinal curvature usually diagnosed during a growth spurt between puberty and the completion of skeletal growth.

Adult scoliosis. A three-dimensional spinal curvature diagnosed after the completion of skeletal growth.

Anterior fusion. A spinal fusion performed through an anterior (front) approach to reach the front of the spine. This approach allows for a stronger fixation of lumbar and thoracolumbar curves. The discs are removed and the spine is fixed.

Boston low profile brace. This is an underarm brace that extends to the hip. It is made from plastic and is designed to fit the patient's needs. Pads are strategically placed on the inside to push on the curves and are usually adjusted monthly.

Cervical vertebrae. The vertebrae of the neck, which are identified as C1 through C7. They connect the neck to the skull at the top and to the thoracic or chest area at the bottom.

Cervico-thoracic. A spinal curvature which has its apex in the region of C7 or T1.

Chronologic age. Age determined by birth date.

Cobb angle. A method of measurement used by physicians to accurately assess the degree of curvature in your spine on an X ray.

Compensatory curve. This is a curve that results from the primary curve, through the body's effort to maintain spinal balance or body alignment. The compensatory curve usually develops above or below the primary curve (major curve).

Congenital scoliosis. A spinal curvature a child is born with, usually secondary to birth defect of the spinal column.

Disc. The portion of the spine located between two vertebrae and characterized as soft and spongy. This portion is usually removed during anterior fusion.

Double major curve. Thoracic and lumbar curves, existing together, generally occurring in opposite directions. Two structural curves.

Functional scoliosis. A curvature that is the result of muscular or gravitational pull on the spine. This curve is nonstructural and usually corrects.

Fusion. The surgical treatment of choice for scoliosis, the goal of which is to fuse the spine into one solid piece, thereby preventing curve progression.

Graft. Bone chips usually taken from the ileum (hindmost pelvic bone) or a rib and implanted in the spine after internal fixation in order to facilitate the spinal fusion.

Idiopathic scoliosis. Scoliosis with no known cause. This type of scoliosis comprises the largest percentage of scoliosis patients and usually manifests during adolescence.

Infantile scoliosis. A three-dimensional curvature of the spine occurring before the age of three.

Instrumentation. Hardware implanted into the spine to decrease curvature and prevent progression. Several different systems are used today.

Kyphosis (roundback). The posterior curve of the spine that is seen from a side view.

Lordosis (swayback). The anterior curve of the lower back that is seen from a side view.

Lumbar vertembrae. The vertebrae in the lower back identified as L1 through L5.

Pseudoarthrosis. A complication of surgery described as failure of the spinal fusion to take place.

Risser sign. A method used to determine bone age based on a scale of one to five, five being fully grown.

Scoliometer. A small, plastic apparatus used by doctors and school nurses to measure discrepancies between elevations of the back by determining the exact degree of spinal rotation.

Structural scoliosis. A three-dimentional curvature of the spine caused by the natural progression of one's spine into a curved position. It persists in the recumbant position.

Thoracic vertebrae. The vertebrae in the upper and mid-back that are identified as T1 through T12. This portion of the spine connects to the neck at the top and to the lower spine (lumbar area) at the bottom.

Notes

1. While many adolescent idiopathic scoliosis (AIS) patients tend not to display any other health problems, the September 1995 *Journal of Musculoskeletal Medicine* included an article titled "Scoliosis: Diagnostic Basics and Therapeutic Choices," which noted that youngsters affected by idiopathic scoliosis may "differ from the general population in their vestibular function, vibratory sensation, growth hormone levels, and skeletal muscle distribution."
2. See chapter 4 for further discussion of subcutaneous rods.
3. J. E. Lonstein and J. M. Carlson, "The prediction of curve progression in untreated idiopathic scoliosis during growth," *J Bone Joint Surg*, 66A: 1061–1071, 1984.
4. My fifteen-year-old brother Blake, on the other hand, does not have scoliosis. While Chloe's spine is curved, and my spine is very curved, Blake's spine is not curved at all! The incidence of scoliosis in my own family is evidence to support the notion that scoliosis is more prevalent in girls.
5. This diagnosis was highly inaccurate. Thirty-degree curves are nowhere near the traditional range of curves that warrant surgery as treatment. At the time of this doctor's visit, though, my mother and I knew nothing more than what the doctor had told us and were both misinformed and devastated.
6. Progression is indicated by the comparison of two X rays over a period of time. For instance, an X ray showing that a patient's spine is curved at a twenty-degree angle and an X ray of the same patient nine months later, illustrating that the spine is curved at a twenty-six-degree angle would be an example of documented progression of the scoliotic curve.
7. Federico P. Girardi and Oheneba Boachie-Adjei, *Clinical Orthopedics*, Philadelphia: J.B. Lippincott, 1999, chapter 31.
8. Note that a lumbar curve can be accompanied by a compensatory thoracic curve. In such a case, the thoracic curve is only present as a result of the lumbar curve, so the lumbar curve will receive more consideration from doctors than the thoracic curve will. Thus, most patients with lumbar curves and compensatory thoracic curves are not considered to have dou-

ble curves (which would necessitate Milwaukee braces); they are customarily treated with Boston braces.

9. Patients with Boston braces need not concern themselves with Charleston braces. Boston braces are meant to be worn during the day and night. The main reason Anthony's doctor suggested use of both braces was that Anthony already a had a Charleston brace in his possession.

10. Although having scoliosis is not synonymous with being crippled (as the name of the hospital implies), Shriners' has an orthopedic unit that has been helpful to many brace-wearing scoliosis patients throughout the years.

11. Sean Barker, "Tennis Star Fights Spine Condition to Standstill," *Connecticut Post*, vol. 6, no. 245, Sept. 2, 1997, p. A1

12. Ibid.

13. Ibid.

14. Letter From Hannah Van Sickle, office of Yo-Yo Ma.

15. Isabella Rossellini, *Some of Me*, New York: Random House, 1997, p. 147.

16. Jesse Kornbluth, "Time Out," *In Style*, June 1997, pp. 152-157.

17. Marian Horosko, "Scuttling Scoliosis," *Dance*, vol. LXV, no. 2, Feb. 1991, pp. 74-75.

18. Ibid.

19. At a check-up during the summer of 1998, my doctor informed me that he thought I did not have to have surgery in December. Hoping to allow me to keep dancing for as long as possible, he has told me that I can wait another few months or years before having surgery. As it stands, both of my curves are hovering in the fifty-degree ranges, I am still dancing, and the date when I will have surgery remains unknown—but it will definitely be within the next two years.

20. While going with the opinion or suggestion that you favor the most may please you or put you at ease, you can never be certain that such an opinion is truly right for you. Your opinion should be reinforced by your research or by other doctors' opinions.

21. See chapter 6 or the glossary for a definition of decompensation.

22. See chapter 8 for a complete definition and explanation of biofeedback.

23. See chapter 6 for the actual percentages and for a more in-depth look at possible complications.

24. See chapter 4 for a closer look at subcutaneous rod systems and their uses.

25. "Anterior Surgery in Scoliosis," *Clinic Orthopedics*, March 1994, pp. 38–44.

26. See chapter 6 for a more detailed description of the crankshaft phenomenon.

27. J. M. Climent, Reiga, J. Sanchez, C. Roda, "Construction and Validation of a Specific Quality of Life Instrument for Adolescents with Spine Deformity," *Spine*, September 1995, p. 2005.

28. Michael Newirth and Kevin Osborn, *The Scoliosis Handbook*. New York: Henry Holt, 1996, pp. 116-117.

29. Oheneba Boachie-Adjei, "Revision Surgery for the Adult Spine Deformity

Patient," *Backtalk*, vol. 21, no. 3, Sept/Oct, 1998.

31. Andrew J. Carr, ChM, FRCS. Consultant Orthopaedic Surgeon, Nuffield Orthopaedic Centre, www.ndos.ox.ac.uk/pcs/index.html

32. Stanley Sacks, "Commentary," *Backtalk*, June/July 1998, vol. 21, no. 2, p. 7.

Index